HELP YOURSELF!

For over three-quarters of a century the Bircher-Benner Clinic of Zurich, Switzerland, has been the center of nutritional treatment of disease. Its staff of physicians and specialists has developed an internationally acclaimed program of meal planning, treatment and physical fitness that is outlined in this series of outstanding health guides.

THE NUTRITION PLAN FOR DIGESTIVE PROBLEMS will aid you in combating a variety of gastrointestinal ailments, including hyper-acidity, colitis, constipation and ulcers. It will show you how to keep your digestive tract strong, stimulated and regular—and offers a versatile dietary program to help you do it.

ABOUT THE BIRCHER-BENNER CLINIC

In the nineteenth century, Dr. M. Bircher-Benner wanted to establish a kind of clinic that had never existed before; a clinic that would take into account the whole man, both body and soul, not only the patient's disease; a clinic that would use an intelligent patient as a co-worker in a total therapeutic effort; a clinic that would use the total knowledge of modern medicine to support the "internal physician"—the autonomous healing forces and healing system of the body—and in every case make the healing effects of dietetic therapy and one's life-style the basis of a total health plan; a clinic that, in addition to eliminating immediate ailments, would bring about a new, tougher, more satisfying and creative health of body and soul for the patient.

The private clinic founded by Dr. Bircher-Benner in 1897 is still operated today for that purpose.

BIRCHER-BENNER

NUTRITION PLAN FOR

DIGESTIVE PROBLEMS

A Comprehensive Guide With Suggestions for Diet Menus and Recipes

Translated by Timothy McManus

By the staff of the Bircher-Benner Clinic:

Medical/Dietetic Section:
D. Liechti-v. Brasch, M.D.,
P. F. Boesch, M.D.,
S. Grieder-Dopheide, M.D.

•

Physiological/Chemical Section:
Alfred Kunz-Bircher, Ph.D.

•

Menus and Recipes:
Ruth Kunz-Bircher, M.D.
(Head of the Bircher-Benner Clinic)

•

Edited by *Ralph Bircher, M.D.*

A JOVE/HBJ BOOK

Published by arrangement with Nash Publishing Corporation

Originally published in Germany under the title *Bircher-Benner Handbuch für Magen und Darmkranke.*

First Jove/HBJ edition published September 1978

Library of Congress Catalog Card Number: 73-186898

Printed in the United States of America

Jove/HBJ books are published by Jove Publications, Inc. (Harcourt Brace Jovanovich) 757 Third Avenue, New York, N.Y. 10017

Contents

I. The Digestive System as Guardian of Health 7
II. Gastric Diseases 13
III. Intestinal Diseases 21
IV. Diets 33
V. Diet Recipes for Gastrointestinal Illnesses . 45
VI. Recipes for Cooked Foods 65
VII. Menu Suggestions 121
VIII. Summary of Food for Various Digestive Ailments 131

I. The Digestive System as Guardian of Health

The stomach and the intestine are given to human beings not only for digesting food and drink. They also form a comprehensive, well structured outwork of the body in its struggle against pathogenic influences in the environment. As long as this outwork is well maintained and ready to function, we are also protected against many dietetic deficiencies and errors. Once weakened or diseased, however, the stomach and the intestine become advanced bases for disease, leaving the body only with limited, inner protection for its defense. Gastrointestinal patients must therefore be very careful in their diet and living habits and must begin to restore healthy digestion if they wish to remain healthy in later years.

The first of these outworks to preserve health is the mouth. It is forgotten all too easily. The mouth is equipped by nature in such a way that it can and should fulfill a number of important tasks in digesting the food. Such tasks are the reduction of food to pulp; salivation for predigestion; and testing the food for its wholesomeness, using the sense of taste to prevent eating unwholesome food, as well as to prepare for absorption and processing in further phases of digestion. This takes place through the secretion of suitable digestive juices throughout the gastrointestinal tract (mouth, stomach, small intestine, liver, pancreas, colon) as soon as the palate detects the taste of the food. When this happens, the digestive system goes into operation. In addition, an array of protective substances (enzymes, antibodies, leucocytes) are available to the healthy digestive apparatus, as soon as the food is in the mouth. Thus, damage from undesirably toxic, infected, denatured, or otherwise upsetting food is prevented or at least reduced.

In many of us, this first outwork, the mouth, is already weak and decaying: food, badly chewed and salivated, is gulped down, and only the most obvious taste stimuli are noticed, while the more delicate individual flavor, which gives information on the real quality of the food, remains unnoticed. Moreover, the response of a palate is drowned out by excessive seasoning and dulled by ingredients that are sharp, far too sweet, irritating, and deadening. While eating, the sick person should concentrate repeatedly on thorough chewing and on the individual taste of each food. As a result of this practice, he will find it intolerable to gulp down such food in large chunks. Correct enjoyment of biting and chewing assures him of a healthy nutritional instinct and a spontaneous aversion to alien, irritating food. The gastrointestinal patient will then understand that he is relieving his digestive organs of a great burden and is contributing considerably to his recovery.

The great observer Traven may not be completely wrong when suggesting a relationship between chewing and human culture: "One has to see the Indian (in southern Mexico) eat, it cannot be described in words. It is music. An attentive grace, a sublime calm guide every movement while eating. We never have time, we have so much to do and yet are never finished. For this reason, we also do not have the time to give to eating the reverence it deserves. We do not eat, we gulp. What took four hours to prepare, we devour in five minutes without thinking. Thus we have civilization, while the Indian has culture."

The mouth is of special significance to human beings, because all its functions are voluntary and hence can be consciously influenced. The rest of the digestive process, on the other hand, happens involuntarily and is much further removed from observation.

Like the mouth, however, the stomach, the duodenum, the small intestine, and the large intestine, as well as all their auxiliary organs, are interconnected outworks of the defense mechanism against disease. With its acids, the stomach disinfects, breaks down and mixes the food, and begins the process of digesting fat and protein.

In conjunction with the liver and pancreas, the duodenum provides for the supply of all necessary, supplementary digestive juices for breaking down and digesting fat, protein, sugar, and starch. It can only fulfill its task correctly, however, if mouth and stomach have adequately prepared the food and if it is consequently able to establish an intestinal environment free of oxygen and bacteria. In the long run, a healthy environment is possible only with the enzymes characteristic of fresh food, avoidance of irritants, and moderation in sugar and meat consumption.

Further digestion takes place in the small intestine. Nutritive substances pass through the portal vein into the liver where more delicate transformation and synthesis take place and existing poisons are rendered harmless. In the lower section of the small intestine and in the colon, the remaining substances are thickened (by the loss of water) and the bacterial destruction of a part of the coarse fibers (cellulose) takes place with the help of digestive bacteria. An intestinal flora assuring full utilization of nutrients thrives in a healthy intestine. It is capable, for example, of producing the important vitamin B_{12}. With healthy food, a well-functioning intestinal environment allows the greatest efficiency in the digestive process and also protects all digestive organs.

The intestinal lining is also an important filter, preventing pathogenic intestinal bacteria and their poisons from entering the bloodstream, while permitting a careful selection of nutritive substances to pass through. If conditions in the intestine are continually unfavorable (*Dysbakteria,* putrefaction, fermentation) the intestinal lining gradually weakens in its power of selection and serious diseases can result from flooding the blood and the whole body with intestinal poison.

To effect a cure, diet is of utmost importance in gastrointestinal disease. It should protect the diseased organs with mechanically prepared food (grated, mashed, pureed, etc.). It must also supply fresh and whole food values, otherwise no prolonged help is obtained. One-sided, strict diets may be supplied for a short time to eliminate acute disturbances, but used too long they often cause new illnesses because they usually lack fresh and supplementary food values.

In this nutrition plan we compiled as many preventive measures as possible known in diet therapy to aid doctor and patient. These are based on the recognition that a sick person is best served by using a diet rich in fresh and whole food values while it protects the weak organs. The condition of the digestive organs makes special adjustments to these diets necessary in individual circumstances. They must sometimes be supplied in the form of juice or puree. Some foods must temporarily be avoided while others must especially be eaten. The aim is to combine medical and dietetic knowledge so that diseased and weakened organs are restored to good health. We would like to emphasize, however, that diet only can in no way replace the advice and treatment of a physician.

II.
Gastric Diseases

Development of the disease. Gastritis can develop slowly and from chronic physical and emotional effects, or it can occur acutely as a result of poisoning or infection. Acute gastritis can quickly be eliminated by strict care and rest, whereas chronic gastritis requires patient and continuous work in order to heal the damage to digestive tissue.

Recurring irritation from food that is too hot, too cold or sharply seasoned, from toxins, lack of fresh food values, prolonged nervous tension, anger, and discontent especially during meal time, causes a *hyperacid, irritated stomach* with artificial hunger pains, sour belching, cramps after eating, heartburn, and soreness when the stomach is empty. Frequent, hasty, excessive, and irritative eating habits, combined with nicotine, alcohol, too much coffee, sweets, aggravate the condition to the point that pain relievers (which are never a cure) are no longer of any help. With prolonged hyperacidity, ulcers requiring clinical care or even surgery can form in such a chronically hyperacid and infected stomach or duodenum.

If the condition of irritation described above persists for very long, the stomach exhausts its digestive juices and slowly becomes a hypoacid slack stomach, which sinks like a lax bag into the intestinal cavity, empties laboriously and slowly, and in which the food begins to decompose if allowed to remain there too long. The results are dull belching, pressure, fullness, flatulence to the point of severe distention, and loss of appetite.

The loss of disinfecting acids allows pathogenic bacteria to penetrate into stomach, intestinal, and bile ducts. Thus infections can develop in the duodenum, liver, gall bladder and colon. Frequent occurrences of fermentative or putrefactive dyspepsia, distention of the abdomen after every meal, constipation and attacks of diarrhea, are the result, since the body's healthy strains of bacteria, necessary for normal digestion, degenerate or die out and are overrun by pathogenic agents. Finally, stomach cancer develops in this environment, as does chronic colitis. If not completely cured, liver diseases (for example, infectious hepatitis) often lead to chronic, hypoacid gastroenteritis. In a gastrointestinal illness, therefore, the liver must be examined thoroughly in order to determine whether any liver damage still exists.

*General guidelines for treatment.** The following principles apply in curing all gastrointestinal illnesses:

Diseased tissue not only requires care, but also new stimulation and training. Every gastrointestinal illness also requires the supply of effective therapeutical ingredients derived from natural raw food: fresh fruit and vegetable juices correctly prepared—the manner of preparation is of special importance. Raw food should be eaten at the beginning of each meal. Moreover, without rest, internal and external relaxation, and an atmosphere of trust and happiness, the gastrointestinal patient cannot recover.

Irritating foods, such as coffee, chocolate, alcoholic beverages, cigarettes and other tobacco products, candy, and sweets are strictly forbidden. Fried and baked foods and white sugar are harmful irritants for an infected stomach.

Slow eating, very thorough chewing (chew every bite as long as necessary until the individual taste of the food, even the after-taste, is noticed), 10 minutes rest before and 30 minutes after each meal must be a strict rule for every gastrointestinal patient in the first weeks of treatment. Notice that efficient operation of the stomach and the intestine depend on good predigestion and secretion of saliva in the mouth and that every hastily chewed or unchewed bit of food unnecessarily burdens further digestion.

In most cases, a few days of complete rest with an appropriate diet is required. Then gradually begin walking exercises. Walking provides the most natural and effective massage and stimulation of digestive organs. It promotes circulation and production of natural juices, peristalsis, and strengthening of tendons. It counteracts enteroptosis and

*For practical suggestions, see "Diets," recipe section and tables.

flatulence in the intestine. The stomach empties properly, and the intestine becomes regular in its functions.

Learn to breathe correctly, especially with the diaphragm and the abdomen. Correct breathing can decisively affect the cure of digestive diseases.

Avoid nervous tension and haste; quiet and relaxation are essential during meals; rest before and after every meal. Retire early at night.

The effect of heat: The hyperacid as well as the hypoacid stomach needs promotion of circulation, warming and relaxation with hot torso packings or compresses. They are wrapped around the abdomen (torso compresses) after eating, or applied as camomile compresses and left on for 20-30 minutes (or as long as they are warm). Moist heat is better than dry heat. Camomile compresses are especially effective. Hot compresses wrapped around the entire abdomen or an electric heating lamp (no sun lamps) are most effective. Depending on the severity of the illness, the patient can lie under the electric heating lamp from one to several hours a day for mild heat (not perspiration) and relaxation.

As soon as warmth is no longer required or agreeable, the stomach patient should switch to the following cold compress: *Torso compress* (after Priessnitx): This compress promotes longlasting, thorough warming of the abdominal region, relaxes cramp feelings, and increases circulation. *Cold* water is best, as it shocks the blood vessels. The cold is counteracted by an increased blood supply in the skin. The warm layer of steam created between the skin and cover has deep reaching effects. The nervous gastrointestinal patient becomes relaxed and drowsy. It is best to apply this compress at lunchtime or at night and to leave it on as long as is agreeable. It is important that the patient feel warm and comfortable before applying this compress. Here's what you do: Dip absorbent cloth (long enough to go around your body) in icy water, wring out, top with thin plastic sheet and immediately place on abdominal region; cover completely with woolen, dry cloth and tighten as much as is comfortable. Upon removal, wash body with cold water.

If available, a connective tissue massage around the stomach can be similarly relaxing and beneficial to circulation, provided it is performed by an experienced, trained hand.

A sluggish intestine in a stomach patient must not be disregarded. Intestinal poisons, especially substances causing putrefaction, enter the bloodstream, strain the healing processes, and cause fatigue, ill humor, and headache. As long as a juice diet is administered, emptying of the intestine should occur two to three times weekly with a camomile enema. Linseed, pureed or finely ground, will later be sufficient. Avoid all chemical laxatives.

Please observe: Every gastrointestinal patient should be under the care of a doctor, who decides whether X-rays or gastric juice testing is necessary. He will tell the patient what kind of stomach trouble he has and how the treatment is to be administered. The patient should furthermore have liver, gallbladder, and pancreas examined.

Treatment of Acute Gastritis

The treatment consists of calming the stomach, uniform warmth, relaxation and tea fasts (Diet I); then a slow transition to a juice diet mixed with pureed cereals, but still containing abundant fresh food values (Diet II A). In this way, the illness is usually overcome in a few days.

Treatment of Chronic Gastritis

1. The Hyperacid Irritated Stomach

This condition requires first an antacid diet with especially mild raw juices, whole grains, puree, absolutely fresh milk, junket, almond milk, and soothing herb teas. Mild raw juices and vegetable juices like carrot, beet, celery root, tomato, and especially cabbage juices (avoid sharp juices from green vegetables like spinach, cress, wild herbs, and radish). By delicately mixing raw juices, all degrees of mildness can be obtained, for example, by adding banana, grape or apple juices to lemon or green juices (see Diet II A, B, page 34). Potato juice, linseed puree, vegetable and animal milk and kaolin are especially antacid. Sour fruit juices (orange, grapefruit, berry, etc.) and juices from green vegetables can be mixed with pureed cereals, agar-agar, cream, and almond milk; whereas mild fruit juices (grape, banana, apple, possibly melon) can be taken plain. After the first and strictest stage of a Juice Diet (Diet II), switch to Pureed Diet (Diet III). White sugar and fried foods must be avoided. From there a slow transition can be made to a Maintenance

Diet, which, carried out for several months, brings about complete recovery of stomach and intestine (Diet IV and V).

Sequence of meals: the irritated, acid stomach should not be overly stimulated with food during the day. Three meals should be enough, allowing the stomach to rest between meals. At most, a few swallows of tea, kaolin, milk, or pureed cereal for calming and natural neutralization of acid can be taken as a snack. Regular consumption of antacid drugs is no remedy; on the contrary, the stomach requires increasingly larger doses and forms larger and larger amounts of acid. Frequent eating to reduce heartburn momentarily is also an ineffective escape. The stomach, hardly through with its work and newly burdened, only increases its acid production and inflammation.

2. The Hypoacid Slack Stomach

Conversely, the slack and hypoacid stomach requires an easy, natural supply of acid and, as soon as feasible, a diet rich in whole grains, raw vegetables, and fruit, in order to help the stomach out of its sluggishness into its own lively movement. First treatment consists again of fresh fruit juices, especially orange, grapefruit, diluted lemon juice, berry juice, sour apples, juices from any vegetables including green leafy ones, wild herbs, white radishes, raw sauerkraut, and cabbage. Fermented milk can also be consumed, such as buttermilk, yogurt, and sour milk (Diet II C).

The soothing addition of pureed cereals and potato juice may also be necessary, since the hypoacid stomach is often sore and inflamed and responds painfully to any strong, irritating taste. As soon as improvement occurs and pressure, fullness, heaviness, and gas decline, turn to a Pureed Diet (Diet III): Muesli made in a blender or passed through a sieve with yogurt, pureed whole-grain cereals, crispbread (well chewed), raw vegetables and fruit prepared in a blender, grated finely or minced. The patient should chew carefully and for a long time, in order to predigest coarse food in the mouth with saliva, and thus to stimulate the sluggish secretion of gastric juices.

Healthy foods that stimulate the secretion of gastric juices and acids: natural vegetable bouillon, yeast extract, herbed cottage cheese, select herb teas (see Types of Tea, page 46), and sour fruit.*

Unhealthy, acid irritants: all roasted products (coffee, roasted meat, fried foods, heated fats), sugar, white flour, alcohol and nicotine.

With a slack stomach, the sequence of meals should also be limited to three main meals, in order to avoid any overloading and to facilitate rest and regeneration between meals. Slight stimulation can be given between meals by a supplement of bitter tea (Wormwood, Centaury, Blessed Thistle—in equal parts), crisp bread, diluted lemon juice or fruit juice, natural vegetable bouillon.

3. Stomach Ulcers

Treatment corresponds largely to Diet II B (in the form of juice and antacid) for hyperacid, irritated stomachs. For a fairly long time, the juices are mixed with one-third pureed cereal or mild vegetable purees. Additional treatment may be necessary, depending on the prescription of a doctor. As early as 1932, Dr. Bircher-Benner reported on the treatment of ulcers with fresh juices. In recent years, results in treating stomach ulcers with large amounts of fresh vegetable juices have been published in America (Cheney, *Management of Gastrointestinal Disorders*, 1950). The therapeutic effect of the "U" factor in cabbage juice, other vegetable juices, and in bananas is now a clinically recognized fact. As a result of these discoveries, drugs have become much less necessary.

One need hardly mention that an ulcer patient requires a greater degree of medical advice and supervision. The development of an ulcer is always the result of many years of a damaging diet and life-style. Without exception, emotional causes are also involved, stemming from years of nervous hypertension, excessive professional stress, dissatisfaction and tension in the home, etc.

The physical (described above) as well as the emotional treatment require serious efforts and patience on the part of doctor and patient, otherwise relapses can be expected. In the case of certain chronic ulcers or excessive tissue formation around the stomach opening, obstructing the functioning and free passage through stomach and intestine, surgery (with frequent dietetic treatment to build up health) is unavoidable.

*See Table II.

III.
Intestinal Diseases

Enteritis, Colitis, Zymosis, Putrefaction

Constipation and diarrhea, the most frequent intestinal maladies, are the expression of a disturbed intestinal function in both the intestinal process as well as the bacterial environment. The patient suffering from an intestinal illness experiences heaviness, fullness, swollen abdomen, difficult bowel movements alternating with colic, and daily attacks of diarrhea and flatulence. Such attacks can occur in apparently rhythmic alternation with constipation after eating certain foods, after irritation, exhaustion, or for no obvious reason; it is the typical picture of enteritis involving the small intestine.

The patient's general condition is influenced as well. He is moody, irritated, and often depressed. He feels tired, tends to have headaches and migraines, and is sensitive to weather. He has poor circulation in hands and feet. A large number of rheumatic patients also suffer from disturbances in the colon (see *Bircher-Benner Arthritis and Rheumatism Nutrition Plan*). When becoming a focus for infection and a source of poisoning, the colon is obviously a burden to total health. If favorable intestinal bacteria are missing, the utilization of food, disposal of waste products and detoxification are disturbed. This also means a lack of antibodies, enzymes, and vitamin complexes (for example, vitamins B_{12}, B_2, and K), which are necessary for correct transformation of food into body cells and energy. Putrefaction and fermentation result in the process (especially if too much was eaten), food left too long in the intestine decomposes, and poisons penetrate into the blood stream through the irritated and weakened intestinal lining and injure body tissue.

The main cause of such disturbed intestinal functions lies in the incorrect diet of the contemporary civilized human being. They are an expression of the general weakening of tissue from a lack of vitally important antibodies and hormones, trace elements, enzymes, and vitamins, that can be assured sufficiently only in a harmonious, well-balanced natural diet. The network of capillaries, the delicately structured and interrelated digestive cells suffer first from dietetic deficiency. Bacteria, given to us for assistance, degenerate and cause disease. Add to that acute, general illness, gastrointestinal-liver infections (hepatitis, enteritis, dysentery, and other tropical diseases when traveling), even a cold, or emotional shock and the result is genuine acute or chronic colitis. Laxatives or congestants are of no help (except for a short period). Neither is a one-sided, strict antacid diet which deprives the organism of the most important nutrients, nor even a change of climate, or scrupulous avoidance of all exertion. Only a return to healthy living and eating habits, and a varied diet that is adjusted to the intestinal condition can bring prolonged help. Morever, there must be no unconscious psychological resistance to a cure.

Severe diarrhea can be treated only under medical supervision, usually in a hospital. After clinical treatment, a chronic intestinal patient is usually able to continue recovery on his own under the supervision of a physician.

General Guidelines for Treatment*

In the therapeutic treatment of intestinal diseases, three forms of diets have repeatedly proved successful.

The raw apple diet (especially in the case of diseases with diarrhea): 2 to 4 pounds of freshly grated apples per day. The lack of protein in this diet removes the breeding ground for bacteria that destroy protein in the intestinal environment. The organic acids of the fruit prevent the growth of these putrefactive agents, and the pectin content of the apples adsorbs the harmful bacterial waste products and prevents their spread into other parts of the body.

The raw food diet (raw vegetables, fresh fruit, and nuts): It contains a great abundance of all vital substances, as well as pectin and cellulose. It also contains the highest concentration of those nutrients not yet fully researched but which are only found in fresh food and which can be of decisive significance in therapy. At the same time, the raw food diet helps to overcome intestinal sluggishness, restore a favor-

*For practical suggestions, see "Diets," recipe section, and tables.

able bacterial flora in the intestine, and to activate the healing process in all body tissues. The preparation of raw foods must be individually adapted (juiced, pureed, or minced; nut or almond milk).

The sour milk diet (yogurt, buttermilk, etc.): It is easily digestible, and is effective because active substances are released in lactic acid fermentation, among which lactic acid itself occurs in the largest amounts. This diet is often especially beneficial to those who have acute and chronic gastrointestinal illnesses, fermentative and putrefactive dyspepsia, meteorism, and chronic constipation.*

Advice on Selecting Food

Starches and Sugar: Potatoes and whole grains are suppliers of starch. Individual preparation can be found in the recipe section. Use only a small amount of sugar mainly in the form of fruit, dried fruit, and honey. White flour, refined sugar, and chocolate should be avoided.

Proteins: High-quality protein is obtained from green leafy vegetables, whole grains, soy products, nuts, milk and eggs. Milk is beneficial when fermented (buttermilk, yogurt, sour milk, junket, whey); casein in the form of cottage cheese, or cream cheese. Sharp and fatty cheeses have an unfavorable effect.

Fats: Restraint in using fats is highly recommended. If possible, use only high-quality fat (obtained by a low-heat process), rich in unsaturated fatty acids, and not overheated in cooking. In addition to cold-pressed vegetable oils (wheat germ, sunflower seed, and corn oils), we also recommend using pure vegetable diet margarines, cream and fresh butter. Avoid fried and baked foods and hydrogenated fats in cooking.

Irritants: Irritants, such as alcoholic beverages, coffee, tea, chocolate, tobacco, strong seasoning (pepper, mustard, salt), and roasted products, must be avoided.

*Pure lactic acid, greatly diluted, functions as an intestinal disinfectant in certain cases. Lactic acid (pure or in sour milk) prevents the growth of unfavorable bacteria, while allowing healthy intestinal bacteria to develop. This effect is also apparent in strong bacterial colonization in the upper section of the small intestine, as microbes disappear and danger of infection in the ascending bile duct is lessened. In diseases of the small intestine and bile duct, this diet is especially important (prepare as in Diet II A, III, and IV).

Food from healthy soil: If food is to be used as a therapeutic remedy, it will be more effective if it is organically grown.

The sluggish intestine needs fresh food in the form of raw vegetables, rich in cellulose and as unreduced in size as possible, fruit and whole-grain dishes. A prolonged and repeated diet of raw foods restores normal intestinal activity and digestion, as well as the intestine's original ability to use food efficiently. The improvement is especially dramatic for the older patient who discovers that the body functions as normally as before on much less food.

With diarrhea, the irritated intestine must be spared as much as possible. Raw food is supplied in the form of juice or puree. Adding vegetable puree to fresh juices makes for even more mildness.

Although diarrhea and constipation are opposite disturbances, they often alternate regularly in the same patient and are both results of prolonged errors in diet, and of deep-seated disturbances in the body's metabolism and detoxification process, with an infection or an emotional conflict often causing the disturbance. Constipation and diarrhea are both expressions of inadequate intestinal movement (slackness or cramping) and disturbed intestinal environments (bacterial infection and poisoning) as a result of which, not only the intestine, but also the liver, pancreas, and stomach suffer and finally the whole organism can become chronically poisoned (rheumatism, migraines, etc.). Both extremes consequently require the same basic principles in treatment: Detoxification, cleansing of the intestine, regulation of digestive processes, as well as one's whole life-style, and particularly, a therapeutic diet of very high quality. Details for adjusting a basic, healthy diet to specific intestinal diseases are cited in Diets I–V, and in the recipe section.

Laxatives: The continuous use of a laxative, even if it works, can in itself never cure. On the other hand, a repeated and prolonged diet of raw food, if rigorously adhered to, almost always leads to normal intestinal activity and digestion, in which nutrients are again fully utilized, and body wastes excreted regularly (see page 43: Maintenance Diet with a Tendency to Constipation).

The intestinal patient needs quiet, relaxed meals and rest and warmth after them. He also needs exercise (walking). The abdominal compress (see page 18) is one of the most valuable aids for stimulation, increasing circulation, and improvement of the intestinal environment. His emotions need serious attention, since for a large number of patients, intestinal disturbances are the clearest expression of severe, unresolved emotional problems.

Intestinal Putrefaction and Fermentation, Intestinal Bacteria

When putrefaction occurs in the intestine, an effort should be made to reduce the protein supply, as for example, with the raw apple diet and the raw food diet. In the case of fermentation, on the other hand, high-quality proteins are used, such as sour milk products, creamed cheeses, soy beans, and the green leaves of raw vegetables and salads. In selecting raw vegetables, choose anti-flatulent ones. They are best administered in the form of juice (Diet II A–C). Grain should be used only finely ground as whole-grain flour, pureed cereal, as crispbread, whole-grain zwieback and sprouted grain bread. Select acid fruits, and those containing little sugar, as for example, berries. Sugar and white flour are to be avoided.

In order to judge the healing process of intestinal diseases, exact bacterial control of the intestinal environment has proved increasingly necessary. In addition to a qualitative and quantitative diagnosis of the intestinal flora, tests are made for pathogenic bacteria, parasites, amoebae, etc., and the degree of fermentation and putrefaction is determined (pH, organic acids, etc.). By supplying normal, living colon bacteria in mouth and intestine, very often a transformation of the intestinal environment is obtained and a more vigorous formation of vital substances results from increased colibacterial growth. For further improving intestinal conditions, an additional supply of vitamins (A, B complex, C) has proved effective, as well as the use of kaolins and vegetable ashes. The doctor may wish to select special herb tea mixtures, which are not cited below. For disinfecting the intestine, it is also possible to use the natural, antibiotic effects of water cress and nasturtium (1/2–1 ounce three times daily). But treatment for infection and parasites must be done by the physician.

Yogurt: In the last 50-60 years, yogurt has been overestimated and underestimated. No therapeutic miracles can be expected from it, but it is neither an unnatural food nor an unhealthy one. Actually, yogurt is, like any other type of sour milk, a food which has been tested the world over, and offered by nature as an available milk food in hot seasons. Yogurt makes an ideal combination with whole grains, potatoes, fresh fruit (or fruit juices), and other foods. Because of its beneficial effect on the intestine, it favorably affects constipation as well as diarrhea and is also nourishing and thirst quenching. Products of lactic acid fermentation are wholesome food and have a dietetic function.

Yogurt is best prepared from boiled milk, since without previous heating a pure yogurt culture cannot be obtained, whereas sour milk, which is raw milk curdled in hot weather, preserves most of the qualities of the raw milk (if it is of faultless quality). Yogurt, sour milk, and buttermilk contain certain lactic acid bacteria, specific to each type of milk mentioned, and, taken moderately, have great healing effects on the bacterial environment of the intestine, promote digestion, and prevent flatulence. They also allow many gastrointestinal patients, allergic to sweet milk (flatulence, cramps, etc.), to consume milk in an acidic form. Pediatricians know the gentle and healing effect of sour milk on the tender digestive system of infants being weaned. Doctors in tropical countries know that a few days of pure buttermilk diet can bring about radical improvement of acute intestinal infection.

Another sour milk product is Kefir, produced by Alta Dena Dairies, which has a yogurt-like taste.

Restraint should be exercised in consuming all types of sour milk. For a sick person's diet, the doctor should give specific directions.

Appendicitis

Such an infection is almost always the result of prolonged irritation of the colon, putrefaction and constipation, caused by an unhealthy diet.

In case of acute pain in the lower abdomen, especially when accompanied by fever, the doctor should always be sent for immediately. Laxatives are strictly forbidden. Abstain from eating and lie still until the doctor comes and decides whether surgery is necessary.

In many cases, chronic appendicitis will require surgery to

achieve a definite cure and to prevent infection from spreading into the body. Often, however, the painful attacks, occurring more or less regularly with chronic appendicitis, are lessened by immediately using a therapeutic diet (complete fast or juice diet). They become less frequent and less severe and heal slowly without surgery. Medical supervision is always advised. Priessnitz compresses applied to the abdomen are soothing.

Gas Formation

This is not a disease in itself, but an extremely annoying, often painful accompanying symptom of chronic gastrointestinal illness. It can occur in connection with a hyperacid, or more often with a hypoacid, stomach, a liver-pancreas disorder, infection of the small intestine, and especially with chronic colitis. Flatulence represents nothing other than the accumulation of gas in the small and large intestines. It is seldom the result of swallowed air (aerophagia), but is a nervous condition produced by feelings of depression, "swallowed anger," and too hasty eating on an irritated stomach. The greater majority of patients suffering from flatulence, have a seriously imbalanced intestinal flora. Many years of inadequate diet, irritating food with the regular addition of sharp seasoning, much salt, coffee, roasted products, sweets, especially alcohol and nicotine, and insufficient exercise and circulation of the abdominal organs are the basis for this degeneration of the intestine. Jaundice or an acute intestinal infection, and especially treatment with antibiotic drugs, some sulfonamides and other disinfectants, can also change the intestinal bacteria. As described earlier, the result is defective production of digestive juices and vitamin deficiency from insufficient utilization of food. Of all these disturbances, the patient often feels only "swelling," flatulence which occurs either after eating or all day long and into the night; it tortures him and, under certain conditions, can degenerate into peritonitis with severe, painful attacks. Often, only special foods cause irregular attacks of flatulence, as for example, hydrogenated fat, refined oils, chocolate, sweet whole milk, cooked cabbage,* fresh bread, certain fruits, sweets, fatty meat, cheese, or hard-boiled eggs. Such individual hypersensitivity to certain foods reveals damage to digestive secretions

*Never flatulent as juice; more flatulent cooked than raw.

or a predominance of special, abnormal or pathogenic strains of bacterial in the intestine. In a specific food environment, these strains of bacteria quickly form gas which can be odorless or intensively sulfurous, depending on the food and type of bacteria. A constipated intestine, whose contents putrefy or ferment, is a storehouse for unfavorable bacteria, and a source of flatulence and of chronic poisons to the blood.

Treatment Guidelines for Meteorism

Overcoming meteorism is achieved by overcoming the basic illness, as described in the individual disease groups. Regeneration of pathogenic intestinal bacteria is achieved as a result of whole food value in the diet and particularly by supplying all antibodies and enzymes, which can only be assured by a natural diet. Denatured food means denatured intestinal bacteria. No disinfectant can bring about a permanent cure when the daily diet does not provide for the correct basis.

As a first step, the intestine should be emptied with a camomile enema or intestinal bath. This should be followed by a day of complete intestinal rest with exclusive consumption of anti-flatulent teas, then transition to a juice diet, followed by a pureed diet. Preference should be given to buttermilk, whey, yogurt, linseed, barley, and rice puree, carrot, beet, and cabbage juice. Several times daily, swallows of raw potato juice, possibly sauerkraut juice, and sea water should be taken. Drink the sour fruit juices mixed with puree; avoid the sweet juices from grapes, sweet plums, peaches, and others, whose high sugar content causes fermentative flatulence. Clean the intestine with camomile enemas every 1-2 days, as long as a juice diet is maintained. The importance of thorough salivation and chewing has already been emphasized. Abdominal compresses and connective tissue massages, as well as breathing exercises, are valuable additional aids (see pages 18-19).

If flatulence is accompanied by diarrhea, the tea day should be followed by an apple day (see Diet II A), possibly also a buttermilk day, especially in summer or in tropical climates. Kaolin with tea for preventing flatulence,* administered between meals, has the effect of absorbing gas and calming the intestine, especially before going to bed at night. Drinking with meals is not beneficial. Raw green leafy vege-

*See Types of Tea, p. 46.

tables are especially valuable, but as experience has shown, they must at first be administered in the form of juice or puree, which is not the case with other raw vegetables. If possible, use organically grown green leafy vegetables. All types of cabbage can be digested as raw juice without causing flatulence. Cooked or raw whole, cabbage is slowly digested and will form gas because of its cellulose content. A continuous supply of whole grain, carefully chewed, will digest well, first as puree, then as sprouted wheat, later as pureed groats and whole-grain bread. Whole grain must replace white flour, small amounts of honey must replace sugar. A little sweet whole milk is allowed only after the first strict transitional diet; sour milk, yogurt, whey, and buttermilk, however, can be drunk before this. Serve teas with lemon juice or some cream instead of with milk. Rest and relaxation before and after meals are important. Emotional problems and professional hypertension are often the main causes of meteorism and prevent normalization of the digestive process. They require attention and resolution. The tendency to become cold must be overcome by exercise, hot and cold showers, dry brushing, etc.

Summary: Meteorism is a result of an unfavorable change in the intestinal bacteria. It can be overcome only by supplying a high amount of fresh raw food in the daily diet and by completely curing chronic constipation. Rest and thorough emptying of the intestine should precede treatment with a therapeutic diet. Denatured, irritating food must be avoided for a long time, intestinal flora must be regenerated, and circulation must be stimulated.

Herter's Disease (Celiac Disease) and Sprue

In 1909, Herter described a children's disease which he called intestinal infantilism, because children afflicted with it were very retarded in their development. Especially striking are the intestinal disorders connected with it, in which the stool with a regular, mixed diet is very abundant, gray, greasy, and soft. A diet rich in starch and sugar causes much gas. The bifidus bacterium prevails, whereas coli and lactic bacteria are missing. The stool occasionally contains a large amount of mucus. Fat, calcium, and magnesium absorption are severely disturbed.

Gluten, a protein present in wheat, rye, oats and barley, is specifically pathogenic because the enzymes necessary to its digestion are lacking. Anemia and vitamin deficiency, caused by diarrhea, are further characteristics of this illness.

Sprue, first observed in the tropics, also occurs in temperate climates and is similar to Herter's disease. It is Herter's disease of the adult, as it were. With regard to therapeutic treatment, it is important that anemia be treated and a gluten-free, carefully combined fresh vegetable diet be administered. Since 1927, when Dr. Bircher-Benner was able to first cure a case of Herter's disease with a raw food diet, some important research results have been obtained. A supply of vitamin E, folic acid, and other vitamins of the B complex promote healing and cause the vitamin E and A content of the blood to rise. Green leaves and vegetables are very important, as well as unsaturated fatty acids in sunflower seeds, wheat germ oil and health food vegetable margarine; also, apples, bananas, strawberries, and blueberries. Because of their gluten content, wheat, rye, barley and oats must be strictly avoided. Other grains and potatoes are digested well and are important because of their vitamin B content. Butter and animal fat intake must be reduced. Since food is poorly utilized in cases of digestive incapacity, all vitally important substances must be administered in carefully balanced meals. Only food of first-rate quality should be selected. Denatured and one-sided foods must be avoided. A supply of protein in the most easily digestible form must be provided: skim milk, whey, buttermilk, cottage cheese and other cheeses made of skim milk; soybeans, almond puree, sesame seed puree, green leaves, and ripe bananas (rich in vitamin E) serve the same purpose. Sugars should only come from natural sources: from fresh fruit, vegetables, well-chewed cereal grains of the types permitted.

Keeping in mind these guidelines, patients afflicted with Herter's disease and sprue must maintain a careful raw food diet, as given under Diets II A and III (see pages 34 and 38). In addition, the patient should occasionally be given vitamin and mineral supplements (calcium, phosphorus, iron, etc.), ultra-violet light baths, and abdominal compresses. Consider also any underlying emotional problems. Every patient with sprue and Herter's disease belongs under the care of a doctor.

IV.
Diets

Diet I. Tea Fast

For acute gastritis and intestinal catarrh, cramps, and febrile digestive illnesses, diarrhea, and mild appendicitis (when surgery can be avoided).

As a pre-treatment for severe meteorism:

> 1-1/2–2 lbs. (3/4-1 qt. tea*) in 5-1/2 oz. glasses, taken in swallows throughout the day. Duration: 1-3 days.

Bed rest, uniform warmth, hot abdominal compresses, Priessnitz compress, camomile enema with 1 qt. camomile tea (repeat 2-3 times until only water comes out).

Diet II. Juice Diet

A. For Acute Enteritis With Diarrhea

The variations in this diet are to be taken on the prescription of a doctor.

One day of Tea Fast is followed by 1 day of apple diet. It provides bulk, cleans, calms, and nourishes with high-quality fresh food, and it is suitable for all types of diarrhea:

Apple day: 1 large, ripe, juicy apple 5-6 times daily (for a total of 2 lbs. apples); peel, liquefy or grate finely, and immediately eat by slow spoonfuls. A few drops of

*Kinds of tea: camomile, linseed, rose hip, marshmallow root, centaury, antiflatulent tea, blueberry, blackberry, and strawberry leaves, unsweetened, with 5-10 drops of lemon juice per glass, see also recipes on pages 46-47.

lemon juice prevent the apple from turning brown. After the first day, 1 ripe banana, thoroughly mashed, can also be mixed with the grated apple. Then change to a pureed diet, observing the guidelines given on page 38.

Or Strawberry day (especially with sprue and chronic enteritis caused by defective fat absorption): 2 lbs. sweet, ripe strawberries without sugar, crushed to a thin pulp with a fork, spread over 5-6 meals. Strawberries are disinfecting and have a special healing effect on sprue and severe infectious diarrhea (typhus and paratyphus). They are rich in vitamins C and A, calcium, potassium, and many other trace elements.

Or Buttermilk day (especially suitable for summer diarrhea in southern and tropical climates where fruit may cause infection): Rapid transformation of intestinal bacterial flora, through non-fat food that is rich in minerals. Can be carried out for a rather long time during hot summer months, possibly alternating with a fresh juice diet: 1 qt. fresh buttermilk, spread throughout the day in 5-6 glassfuls. No additional food should be taken except for herb tea.

Or Juices with pureed cereal (with diarrhea after an Apple day, or after a day of Tea Fast): Mix juices with 1/3 rice or barley puree or a little cream. Especially effective against diarrhea are juiced or pureed blueberries, grapefruit, strawberries, black currants, grated apples and mashed bananas blended with other fruit juices. Juices of pitted fruits should be used only after diarrhea has stopped.

Vegetable juices: carrot, beet, tomato, cabbage, celery and celeriac, Boston lettuce. In the beginning avoid spinach, white radish, cress, onions, garlic, and sauerkraut. *Milk:* buttermilk, mild whey, health food store low-fat yogurt, very diluted almond and soybean milks.

For a sample Daily Menu see page 40.

For thirst quenching (patients with diarrhea suffer strongly from thirst): strawberry, blueberry, and blackberry leaf tea, peppermint tea, camomile tea (possibly anti-flatulent tea).

Black tea must be avoided because of its theine content and its insomniac effect.

General treatment for acute enteritis: Camomile enema with 1 qt. camomile tea and 1 tbsp. kaolin, every 2 days. Hot compresses for cramps; abdominal compress at night. Continue bed rest as long as fever and diarrhea persist.

B. For A Hyperacid Stomach, Ulcers

Bed-Juice Fast

After 1 day of Tea Fast, or to begin with: 21-28 oz. fresh fruit and vegetables juices, throughout the day for 2-3 days (mixed with pureed cereal, if necessary). If possible, use organically grown food.

Fruit juices: Oranges (if no hypersensitivity exists), grapefruit, tangerines, grapes, berries, apples, peaches, sweet plums, melons, cherries—freshly pressed and mixed with 1/3 pureed cereal (linseed, rice, barley), cream, and agar-agar. Omit sweet types of fruit in cases of strong meteorism.

Vegetable juices: carrots, beets, tomatoes, lettuce, spinach, cress (in spoonfuls as soon as digestible), celery and celeriac, fennel, white radish—freshly pressed and mixed with 1/3 pureed cereal, agar-agar, or 1/3 cream, as with fruit juices. Plus 4 oz. cabbage juice daily (from organically grown cabbage) with 2 oz. of potato juice pure or mixed with other juices.

Linseed puree: 2-5 cups in swallows, throughout the day. For preparation of purees, see recipes (page 49).

For heartburn, use kaolin and camomile tea, 1 tsp. 3-5 times daily. Other remedies should be prescribed by a physician. We do recommend *nux vomica* as a very effective homeopathic remedy against cramps. Use 8 drops 3-6 times daily.

Full Juice Fast Diet

A Full Juice Fast diet of 2-7 days follows 2-3 days of a Bed-Juice Fast. In addition to the fresh juices mentioned, the following are administered: almond milk,* mild fresh yogurt,

*Almonds, finely ground, well chewed, or as milk, have a soothing, curative effect on the stomach lining. Unlike drugs they are a natural antacid.

or certified milk (if tolerated), junket, sesame or soybean milk, mild, fresh buttermilk, whey.

Example of a Daily Menu

Morning and
Evening: 7 oz. mixture of fruit juice and pureed cereal or cream, 5½ oz. almond or soybean milk or agar-agar, 5½ oz. mixture of fruit juice and cream, 5½ oz. mild yogurt.

Noon: 7 oz. mixture of fruit or vegetable juice, 5½ oz. buttermilk or whey† or yogurt or certified milk. Cabbage and potato juice once daily, 5½ oz. Linseed puree at night, in case of pain.

For thirst: Teas described under Diet I. Noncarbonated mineral water (the doctor should select the type).

General treatment: Predominantly bed rest, hot compresses after eating. After good initial pre-warming, an abdominal compress for the night, applied cold. Relaxation. Breathing exercises. 1 qt. camomile enema every 2 days. For heartburn, kaolin with camomile tea between meals plus 1 tsp. 3 times in the evening.

C. For A Hypoacid Stomach

After 1 day of Tea Fast, or to begin with: 2-3 days of a Full Juice Fast diet. Fruit and raw vegetable juices as described in Diet II B, but without the addition of pureed cereal: Grapefruit, orange, diluted lemon juice, berries of any kind, sour apples, ripe pitted fruit; spinach, white radish, sauerkraut, sauerkraut water, sea water, lettuce, other raw vegetables.

Milk: sour milk, yogurt, sour buttermilk, whey. Sweet whole milk is usually poorly digested (fullness, flatulence): salivate and warm in the mouth before swallowing.

If in rare cases a hypoacid stomach is so irritated that it in-

†Whey is the liquid residue after milk has been coagulated, consisting of sugars and minerals, and vitamins in the milk, a nonfat, easily digestible, and high quality beverage—extra alkaline.

itially reacts to sour juices with discomfort, you can add ⅓ pureed cereal, especially linseed puree (mixed with the juices, or taken a little at a time, alternately with the juices). This will also be slightly laxative and stimulate peristalsis.

Example of a Daily Menu

Morning: 7 oz. fruit juice, 5½ oz. yogurt or buttermilk.

Noon: 5½ oz. fruit juice, 5½ oz. vegetable juice, 5½ oz. yogurt or buttermilk or sour milk.

Evening: 7 oz. fruit or vegetable juice, 5½ oz. yogurt or buttermilk.

For thirst: Acidifying types of tea like "bitter tea" (wormwood, centaury, blessed thistle in equal parts), juniper juice (in spoonfuls), marshmallow, centaury, peppermint, yarrow.

Acidifying vegetable broth with stimulating herbs, yeast, and soy sauce for seasoning: 1-2 cups per day. Carbonated mineral water. Water or sea water with lemon juice, but without sugar.

General treatment: Eat slowly and salivate the juices well. Regular rest before meals, a short rest in the afternoon. In addition, walking, light exercises (for abdominal muscles), abdominal massage with a vibrator, connective tissue massage around the stomach, hot and cold water treatment for the abdomen, or hot abdominal compresses with a final cold washing. Apply compresses in the evening after first getting warmed up by walking. Take 1 tsp. kaolin 3 times during the day for flatulence. Do not let constipation linger. Use a camomile enema every 2 days as long as a juice diet is maintained.

Diet III. Pureed Diet

After Diet II is concluded, a pureed diet is used for both a hyperacid and hypoacid stomach, after stomach operations, and after enteritis. This diet is a slow transition to solid food. It should contain all important nutrients properly balanced, permit no deficiencies especially when carried out for a long time; satisfy the appetite and complete healing with an economic supply of food. It is therefore a complete diet, but still specially prepared. It can be easily adjusted to the patient who is sensitive to fat, animal protein, and milk, or who has a strong need for milk casein protein; as well as to the patient with a sensitivity to certain fruits and vegetables (onions, etc.), a tendency to flatulence or a deficiency of vitamins C or B.

Such sensitivity is often overestimated and a number of foods and combinations are anxiously avoided. Several different and conflicting dietetic theories place great importance on such rules. We shall see again and again, however, that such sensitivity disappears slowly and surely with correct eating and that the patient will come to have the full choice of healthy foods needed by his body. However, especially in the beginning, scrupulous adjustment to individual reactions is indicated.

Dietetic Guidelines

Fresh Fruit: apples, peaches, melons, etc., bananas, berries, unheated and as fresh as possible, grated or mashed. Cooked fruit does not replace fresh fruit and should only be eaten occasionally.

Fresh Vegetables: pureed raw in a blender or minced, mixed and seasoned very lightly with cream, oil, lemon juice, and almond puree (see Salad Dressings). Raw cabbage, except as juice, should still be avoided. Serve vegetables immediately after they have been prepared. Cooked vegetables (including cabbage, page 85) should be strained (sieve or blender).

Milk: all types, plain if digestible, plain or in salads, fruits, soups, and muesli. Yogurt and buttermilk take preference over sweet, whole milk. Also soybean, almond, and sesame milk, whey. Milk products: cottage cheese mixed, if needed, with herbs and acidifiers (yeast extract, soy, and other similar seasonings) plain, or with fruit juice and honey. Cream cheese and other soft cheeses, but no fat, cooked cheeses. Sunflower seed oil.

Sweeteners: fruit concentrate, sweet fruit juices, a little honey, no white sugar.

Grain: only whole grain, as pureed brown rice, barley,

oats, wheat, as flour, as cooked puree of groats, as soup (oat, barley, rice, wheat), as crispbread (well chewed), or as dietetic zwieback.

Potatoes: in their jackets, or mashed, never fried.

Fats: cold-pressed high-quality vegetable oils, especially sunflower seed, corn, olive, and wheat germ oils. Slowly increase consumption of fresh butter, on bread and in cooked dishes. Cream in muesli and soups. Health food store vegetable fats for cooking and spreads. Do not use heated or hydrogenated fats.

Eggs: fresh raw egg 2-3 times a week in juice, vegetable broth, and soup, if tolerated.

Beverages: all herb teas mentioned in Diet II A–C, mineral water and fresh juices according to need.

Meat: see page 43.

Avoid: alcohol, tobacco, coffee, white sugar, white flour, mustard, pepper, curry, hot sauces, fried, roasted, breaded foods.

Strain everything, and salivate well.

Example of a Daily Menu

Morning: Bircher muesli with yogurt in a blender or cereal soup and fruit
fruit juice with cream, crispbread with butter and honey or cottage cheese. Herb tea.

Noon: Mashed bananas and oranges with some cream or almond milk
2-3 raw vegetables combined in a blender
mashed potatoes
strained cooked vegetables, mineral water
compote or fruit gelatin.

Evening: Blender muesli or yogurt and fruit juice or junket and fruit juice
cereal soup or porridge or vegetable broth (plain or mixed with 1 egg) and 1 baked potato. Herb tea.

Between meals: If thirsty, tea, fruit juice, buttermilk, or yogurt, possibly cottage cheese.

General treatment: as in Diets A, B, C.

Example of a Daily Menu

(For patients of sprue and Herter's disease following Juice Diet II A)

Morning and
Evening: Bircher muesli blended with unsweetened condensed milk
1 glass almond milk
1 mashed banana with cottage cheese, 1 tsp. linseed oil, diet bread (no wheat, rye, barley, oats).

Noon: 1 grated apple, possibly 1 mashed banana
mixed raw salad, dressed with cold-pressed linseed oil and lemon juice
soup of pureed brown rice, millet, or soy flakes (but not oats, barley, wheat or rye), or mashed potatoes or linseed puree, carob bread.

Afternoon
snack: Carob bread or grated apples or mashed bananas and soybean flakes
camomile tea (if thirsty).

General treatment: Abdominal compresses, ultra-violet light bath.

Diet IV. Transition Diet

After concluding Diet III, a transitional diet is indicated for 2-3 months of convalescence from gastrointestinal illness, for chronic, mild enteritis, food sensitivity and a "sensitive" stomach.

This diet corresponds extensively to the normal Bircher-Benner diet, but still requires food carefully prepared, selectively combined and of especially high quality. Never overeat. Moderation often plays a decisive role in healing an injured gastrointestinal tract. Thorough chewing at meals and attention to taste will help rediscover the natural sense of selection and a feeling of satiety so that excessive and indigestible food can be avoided automatically. The transitional diet should be simple and should avoid too great a variety of foods in the same meal, complicated dishes, sauces, etc. It no longer emphasizes care and protection, but seeks to develop the instinctive appreciation of wholesome food, and to strengthen restored health.

If recovery from a gastrointestinal illness fulfills a purpose, it is that suffering and restrictions add to personal experience, i.e., to regain insight and self-control, and to learn to enjoy healthy pleasures and activities which enrich personal development and maturity. Convalescence from a gastrointestinal illness depends not only on diet, but also on the solution of emotional causes responsible for the disease. Very often, the tranquility required by the illness gives strength and time to understand and overcome anxiety, uncertainty, a repressed fear or guilt.

Dietetic Guidelines

Simple preparation. Only 1 kind of fruit and 1-2 kinds of fresh vegetables (salads), 1-2 cooked vegetables during the same meal. Only exceptionally serve: baked dishes, brown gravies, sauteed onions, mayonnaise, French fries. Irritants such as roasted, baked, and fried foods, chocolate, coffee, tea, sweets, alcohol, and nicotine should not be touched. Have three meals per day, snacks only as an exception. Allow the foods to be as natural as possible.

Fruit and fresh vegetables: every kind and combination, when necessary, still very finely chopped, avoiding strong herb seasonings on salads (or serve only as an exception). Preference should be given to very fresh and ripe fruit, and organically grown fresh vegetables whenever possible.

Cooked vegetables: steam only in very little water. Use sea salt instead of table salt and vegetable broth instead of water. Cooked cabbages are much harder to digest than raw cabbages. Leave vegetables as natural as possible, simply prepared, without gravies and onions.

Potato dishes: plain, mashed, or whole, not fried.

Grain dishes: crispbread (such as Ry-Krisp, Wasabröd), pumpernickel, diet zwieback. Semolina, cornstarch, and sago are used only as thickening agents. Use corn, millet, barley, oats, and brown rice for soups or porridge (with flakes or groats). White flour or noodles and other such products should not be used more than once a week.

Eggs: in any form, but not more than 2-3 per week, preferably raw.

Fats: preferably vegetable oils with a high content of

highly unsaturated fatty acids (linoleic acids), linseed oil, sunflower seed oil, fresh butter and cream. Baking, roasting and heated fat must be avoided.

Milk and milk products, as well as beverages: as in Diet III.

Meat: only as an exception, if desired. From an experience, the desire for meat usually diminishes if the palate and the whole digestive tract become accustomed to natural and harmonious food that is free of irritants.

Diet V. Maintenance Diet

As an expansion of Transition Diet IV, it is a healthy, basic diet, intended to prevent recurrence of ailments.

This diet corresponds extensively to Diet IV, but is less rigid, and allows more variation.

Crispbread, whole-grain porridge, cracked grains (groats), and sprouted grains are allowed as whole-grain nourishment.

For variety, complex dishes, baked puddings, dessert creams, sauces, rice dishes and meat (if desired) can occasionally be enjoyed, 1-2 times weekly.

The guidelines for the diet, however, remain simple and as a rule, natural dishes are always preferable to denatured food.

Alcohol, white flour products, habitual use of coffee and nicotine should be avoided in the long run. In this way, the healthy stomach and intestinal environment remain intact and relapses are avoided.

Maintenance Diet in the Case of a Tendency to Constipation

With chronic constipation, a complete and permanent diet is required. No laxatives (including cigarettes, and morning coffee) please. The sluggish intestine must be given the time and opportunity to retain itself. It must not be supported in its sluggishness by giving it a constant helping hand with chemical "boosts." The simplest and quickest way to achieve the goal is to convert to a pure raw food diet for 1-3 weeks. Usually a week is sufficient to produce a far-reaching change in the intestinal environment and natural peristalsis in the colon. In the raw food diet, unnatural irritants are automatically eliminated. Try to maintain a regular daily schedule, get sufficient sleep and exercise (walking, stimulation of abdominal muscles and intestine by massage, gymnastics, hot and cold showers, dry brushing). If one week of a Raw Food Diet is not sufficient to cure many years of constipation, the patient should hold out for 2-3 weeks, until the intestine empties easily and completely by itself, 1-3 times daily. With persistence, the goal is almost always attained. 1-2 tbsp. of linseed flour, or linseed tea, also dried fruit, rhubarb, raw or cooked, wheat groats may be of added assistance.

As soon as constipation is overcome, carefully switch from a raw diet to a high-quality normal diet (Diets IV, V), strictly avoiding white bread, white flour, white sugar, chocolate, coffee, and alcohol for months. A raw diet should be included 1-2 days per week for safety. Do not forget to chew well, eat slowly, get fresh air and exercise.

Chronic constipation results in widening of the colon and infection, hemorrhoids, anal fissures, cramps in the sphincter muscle. These symptoms complicate healing of constipation and require medical supervision and care.

Example of a Raw Diet Day

(Prolonged diet of 2-3 weeks for constipation)

Morning: Bircher muesli of mixed fruit with yogurt or condensed milk or fresh grain mash with yogurt and fruit
herb tea with 1 tsp. honey
sprouted wheat, nuts, dried fruit.

Noon: Various fruits
3 different salads (many green leaves)
dried fruit, nuts, sprouted grains
buttermilk or natural, organic apple juice.

Evening: As in the morning, but possibly instead of muesli, junket or yogurt with Kellogg's "All Bran" (or similar bran cereal), dried fruit
fresh fruit.

When changing to a normal diet, whole-grain bread, butter, steamed vegetables, potatoes, and grain dishes can be used as a supplement.

V.
Diet Recipes for Gastrointestinal Illnesses

Types of Tea

1. Camomile Tea

Steep only. Drink for abdominal pains (has a cleaning and calming effect on the gastrointestinal tract). For enemas and infusions.

2. Peppermint Tea

Steep only. Calming, choleretic, stimulates small intestine.

3. Lemon Verbena Tea

Steep only. Calming, reduces phlegm, choleretic. Afternoons and evenings.

4. Yarrow Tea

Prepare like camomile tea. Stimulates stomach, spasmolytic, heals infection, stops bleeding.

5. Strawberry Leaf Tea

Prepare like peppermint tea. Slightly constipating.

6. Blackberry Leaf Tea

Prepare like peppermint tea. Slightly constipating.

7. Seed Tea

Caraway seed, fennel, anise in equal parts. Steep and leave for 20 minutes. For flatulence: drink 1 full cup after meals.

8. Bitter Tea

Wormwood, centaury, blessed thistle (equal parts). Steep and leave for 5 minutes. With loss of appetite, drink 2-3 tbsp. 1/2 hr. before meals. Slightly choleretic, stimulates digestive juices. For sensitive patients: only centaury tea, prepare like camomile tea.

9. Rose Hip Tea

Soak 2-3 tbsp. rose hip seeds and shells for 12 hrs. in 1-1/2 qt. water, then boil gently 1/2–3/4 hr., strain. The remaining rose hips can be boiled again with fresh rose hips on the following day. Slightly choleretic and diuretic, refreshing, stimulating.

10. Linseed Tea

Boil 1 tbsp. 7-10 minutes in 1/2 qt. water and let steep. Mucolytic, slightly laxative, calms stomach.

11. Marshmallow Root Tea

1 tbsp. to 1/4 qt. water, boil 5 minutes, steep 10 minutes, strain. Cleans stomach and intestine and calms.

12. Blueberry Tea

Soak 1 tbsp. dried blueberries 12 hrs. and boil 5 minutes. Strain. Constipating, calming.

Juices and Cereal Purees

Juices*

Raw food in mechanically refined form as an additional

*When it is impossible to prepare juices yourself, high-quality bottled grapefruit and vegetable juices can be obtained from a health food store.

special enrichment and when bulk (cellulose) is forbidden.

Do not forget, however, that whole fresh food is more valuable and cannot be replaced by juices for a long period. Therefore, return to fruit and raw vegetables as soon as possible.

For cleaning, see the chapter on "Raw Vegetables." For preparing fruit and raw juices many presses are on the market, from the small hand press to the electric juicer. If a hand press is used, fruit and vegetables must be reduced in size.

Grate finely apples, pears, and all tuberous vegetables, chop finely all leafy vegetables and herbs.

13. Fruit Juices

Serve immediately after pressing. Letting them stand means a loss in value.

a) Plain fruit juices (without any supplement):
oranges, tangerines, grapefruit, apples, pears, grapes, strawberries, blueberries, currants, raspberries, peaches, apricots, sweet plums, melons, cherries

b) Mixed fruit juices (only citrus fruit, if tolerated):
oranges, tangerines, grapefruit, possibly Japanese persimmons
or berry juice with apple juice
or berry juice with peach, apricot, or plum juice
mashed bananas with orange, berry, peach, and apricot juice

Depending on desire or prescription, add: Lemon juice, raw sugar, honey, fruit concentrate, cream, yogurt, almond milk, linseed, rice, or barley puree, wheat gel.

14. Vegetable Juices

High mineral and vitamin content when freshly pressed. Each juice has its own nutritional value (see chapter on minerals and vitamins in the Bircher-Benner cookbook, *Eating Your Way to Health*, published by Penguin Books).

a) Unmixed Vegetable Juices:
tomatoes, carrots, beets, white radish, cabbage, celery, potatoes, all leafy, tuberous, and root vegetables

b) Mixed Vegetable Juices:
carrots, tomatoes, spinach (equal parts)
tomatoes and carrots
tomatoes and spinach

In our experience, these are the best mixtures. Other mixtures (and cocktails) can be combined according to individual taste.

For a change, add before extracting: sorrel, stinging nettle, chives, parsley, onions, tender celery leaves or roots and other herbs.

Add per glass (6-8 oz.): 1 tsp. cream, some lemon juice, possibly some fruit concentrate, possibly linseed, rice, or barley puree. Other leafy vegetables or lettuces can also be used, for example, white cabbage, savoy cabbage, endive, salad-bowl lettuce, Romaine lettuce, dandelion. In the spring, purify the blood with the juice of stinging nettle, sorrel, and dandelion.

c) Potato Juice:
Use well cleaned, possibly peeled potatoes (no unripe or sprouted potatoes with green spots).
Prepare like carrot juice. Taste is not very pleasant. On doctor's prescription before meals (spasmolytic, healing).

15. Cereal Puree as a Supplement to Juices

Mix with raw juices up to 1/3 the amount; neutralizes the sharpness of the fruit taste.

a) Rice or Barley Puree:
1 heaping tsp. rice or barley meal
1/5 qt. water

Stir cereal into cold water and boil for 5 minutes while stirring. Let cool.

b) Linseed Puree:
   1 tbsp. linseed
   1/5 qt. water

Wash seeds and boil in water for 10 minutes, strain, and let cool.

The daily amount can be prepared once a day, stored in a thermos bottle and added to each freshly prepared raw juice as required.

Types of Milk

16. Almond Milk

(Vegetable protein-fat-food, reduces phlegm, soothing)

1 tbsp. almond mash
1 tsp. honey
12 tbsp. water
or
12 tbsp. water with 4 tbsp. fruit juice to produce a slight thickening

Mix almond mash and honey with a whisk and add the water drop by drop.

17. Almond Milk from Fresh Almonds

(Very digestible)

1-1/2 tbsp. shelled almonds
1 tsp. honey
12 tbsp. water

Mix almonds, honey and water in a blender, possibly strain. Do not use bitter almonds.

18. Pine Kernel Milk

(Very rich in easily digestible fat and vegetable protein)

1-1/2 tbsp. washed pine kernels

1 tsp. honey
12 tbsp. water

Prepare like almond milk.

19. Sesame Seed Milk

1/5 qt. water (cold or warm—depending on taste)
1 level tbsp. sesame puree
1 tsp. raw sugar or honey

Mix sesame puree and sugar or honey with a whisk and add the water drop by drop.

20. Soybean Milk

Wash and dry soybeans, crush in an almond mill.

1 cup soybeans
7 cups water
2 tbsp. sugar

Soak soybeans for 2 hrs., then boil for 20 minutes in the soaking water while stirring constantly. Strain, add water until mixture has the consistency of regular milk. Add sugar, let cool.

21. Yogurt

Yogurt is a pure and easily digestible form of milk protein, promotes digestion.

You can make yogurt yourself in a yogurt maker or buy it in the health food stores.

22. Junket* with Fruit

3/4 qt. milk
1-2 tbsp. raw sugar
Vanilla sugar or grated lemon peel
1/2 junket tablet
1 tbsp. water

*Junket, a product of lightly soured milk, is available in tablets in better health food stores; it is imported from England.

Fresh sugared berries
8 tbsp. heavy cream

Warm the milk with the flavoring and honey to about 98 degrees F. Crush the tablet and dissolve in water, then place in the warm milk, stir quickly and immediately pour into glasses. Let the junket set and cool. Sprinkle the berries over the junket shortly before serving and garnish with whipped cream.

Bircher Muesli

The original apple muesli, as first introduced by Dr. Bircher, has remained one of the best diet foods in our long years of experience.

Sour, white-fleshed, juicy apples are best, for example, Pippin, Golden Delicious, Jonathan, Ontario, Wellington.

If apples are dry or tasteless, the flavor can be improved by adding some freshly grated orange or lemon peel or orange juice, or occasionally some rose hip puree just before serving.

If allowed by the physician, add high quality sugar, honey, nuts to any muesli. *Never* in the acute stage of a gastrointestinal illness.

23. Apple Muesli

1 level tbsp. rolled oats
3 tbsp. cold water
1 tbsp. lemon juice
1 tbsp. condensed milk, unsweetened, possibly 1-2 tbsp. water, depending on the kind of apple
7 oz. apples
1 tbsp. hazelnuts (filberts) or almonds, grated

Soak oats for 12 hours in water. (Do not soak instant oats. The amount of water remains the same, however.) Blend oats, lemon juice and condensed milk into a smooth puree. Wash apples, dry with a clean cloth, remove stem and core. Just before serving, grate the apples directly into the puree, stirring often to prevent discoloring. Sweeten with half a banana, honey, fruit concentrate or other natural sweeteners. Sprinkle with filberts.

Instead of 1 tbsp. rolled oats the following can be used: 1 tsp. rolled oats, soaked, and 1 tsp. cereal grains. Soak the grains in water 24 hrs., spread on sieve and rinse with cold water, then add whole, crushed, or mixed in blender.

Rolled wheat, rice, barley, rye, millet, buckwheat, or soy-flakes can also be used, or dried, crushed wheat flakes available in health food stores, possibly mixed with yeast flakes (rich in vitamin B).

24. Apple Muesli with Almond Puree

A diet when animal protein is forbidden (allergies).

1 level tbsp. rolled oats
3 tbsp. water
1 tbsp. lemon juice
1 tbsp. almond puree
1 tbsp. honey or raw sugar
3 tbsp. water
7 oz. apples
1 tbsp. grated almonds

Soak oats in water for 12 hrs. Mix all ingredients except apples thoroughly with a whisk. Prepare apples as in basic recipe No. 23. Sprinkle dish with grated nuts.

25. Apple Muesli with Yogurt

A diet when milk is indigestible—promotes digestion strongly, is less filling and more tart than milk.

1 level tbsp. rolled oats
3 tbsp. water
3 tbsp. yogurt
1 tsp. lemon juice
1 tbsp. honey or 1-1/2 tbsp. raw sugar
7 oz. apples
1 tbsp. grated almonds

Soak oats in water for 12 hours. Blend all ingredients except apples into a smooth puree. Prepare apples like basic recipe No. 23. Sprinkle nuts over the prepared dish.

26. Apple Muesli with Cream

Specially enriched dish if an increase in weight is desired.

1 tsp. rolled oats
1-2 tbsp. water
3-4 tbsp. cream
1 tsp. lemon juice
1 tbsp. honey
7 oz. apples
1 tbsp. grated almonds

Soak oats in water for 12 hrs. Whip cream slightly and mix with the lemon juice and honey. Prepare apples as in basic recipe No. 23. Sprinkle nuts over the prepared dish.

27. Muesli with Berries or Pitted Fruit

Especially high vitamin C content.

5-1/2–7 oz. washed choice strawberries or raspberries, blueberries, currants, blackberries or plums, apricots, or peaches.

Squash berries with a fork or pestle. Put pitted fruit through a chrome-plated chopper or mince with a knife.

28. Muesli with Assorted Fruit

Strawberries and raspberries
Strawberries, raspberries, and currants
Strawberries and apples
Blackberries and apples
Apples with thin slices of oranges and tangerines
Apples and bananas

(To prepare the puree, see basic recipe No. 23.)

Note: Depending on the condition of the stomach or intestine, all recipes can be finely pureed in a blender. Follow the advice of a doctor.

Raw Vegetables

In preparing raw vegetables, observe the following basic principles:

1. Freshness

Sun-ripened, organically grown vegetables are best, out of your own garden or from the health food store.

Prepare raw vegetables as shortly as possible before serving to prevent wilting or loss of juice. Mix quickly with dressing so that the crushed or sliced food is only briefly exposed to the air.

2. Quality

Leafy and root vegetables should be young, tender, organically grown and free from plant diseases. This is especially important for an invalid diet.

3. Cleanliness

Follow the instructions below for cleaning vegetables exactly to avoid infection with colibacilli.

Properly composted vegetables (no animal manure) contain no worm eggs.

4. Harmony

Whenever possible, a raw salad dish should consist of tuberous-fruit-leafy vegetables. The green leafy vegetable should never be missing from a sick person's diet. There should also be variation in the dressing for the same raw salad.

A trio of colors make the dish attractive and contribute to enjoyable eating.

Small garnishes of herbs, radishes, and new carrots, etc., can colorfully and festively decorate a salad on special occasions, but three raw vegetables per meal should not be exceeded, variety being provided at other meals. Excessive variety does not benefit digestion. This last means: not too much variety at any one meal.

Cleaning Leafy Vegetables

Boston lettuce, endive, Romaine lettuce, white cabbage, red cabbage, etc. Separate the leaves, remove brown and damaged spots, and soak for 1 hour in salted water (1 handful to 5 qt. water). Rinse several times—it is best to rinse every leaf individually under running water. Shake in a wire basket or in a clean cloth to dry.

Leaf lettuce and loose-leaved lettuce, spinach, dandelion, cress, Brussels sprouts, and similar small leafy lettuces require special care in separating and washing. Rinse several times in small amounts, remove roots and tough stalks.

Cut Belgian endive in half, remove outermost leaves and rinse well.

Cleaning Tuberous Vegetables

Celery root (celeriac), carrots, salsify, beets, white radish, kohlrabi, and radishes. Clean the roots with a brush under running water. Peel and place immediately in cold water mixed with salt and lemon juice (1/2 lemon or left-over peel to 5 qt. water), so that the vegetables retain their fresh color.

Cleaning Fruit Vegetables

Tomatoes, cucumbers, zucchini, bell pepper. Wash the fruit first, then possibly peel or cut into small pieces. Peel cucumbers from the center outwards, cutting off the bitter ends. Tender cucumbers can also be used unpeeled. For salads, use only young, tender zucchini, unpeeled. Green and yellow bell peppers are less sharp than red ones. Cut the peppers in half and remove seeds and thick stems, and possibly soak in water, if too sharp.

Cauliflower, celery stalks, leeks, fennel. Cut the cauliflower into rather large pieces, cut away damaged spots, peel large stem, and soak in salt water. Peel celery stalks, cut away tough parts. Cut leeks in half, prepare, and wash under the tap. Cut fennel in half and wash.

Special Cleaning Methods

Should there be any doubts about the cleanliness and

freedom from germs of vegetables, and possibly also fruit (especially in southern and tropical countries), observe the following cleaning methods:

Place the vegetables in a diluted table salt solution (1 handful of salt to 5 qt. water).

Bacteria, colibacilli, and mold, while of no danger to healthy people in temperate climates, can be removed with citric acid and vinegar. Make a solution of 2 oz. citric acid (available at the drug store) with 1 qt. water and soak vegetables, especially leafy ones, for 15 minutes. Then rinse well under running water. Save the citric acid solution; it can be reused 3-4 times.

After cleaning, tuberous and fruit vegetables can be placed in a colander or wire basket and dipped in boiling water for about 10 seconds. In the process, the outer layer becomes germ free and the vegetable still remains raw on the inside.

Vegetable and fruit juices can be made almost germ free if fresh lemon juice is added to 3/5 of the amount of juice.

In order to guard against amoebic infection in the tropics, dip the prepared vegetables in a calcium chloride solution (1/5 oz. calcium chloride to 1 qt. water). Then wash in boiling water, in which the calcium chloride is completely removed.

Preparation of Various Vegetables

Boston lettuce, loose-leaved lettuce, leaf lettuce, dandelion, cress—Leave whole or cut the largest leaves in half.

Romaine lettuce, endive, Belgian endive—Cut into strips 1/4 in. wide.

Spinach, leek, bell pepper, celery stalk, fennel—Cut into very thin strips.

Cabbage, white cabbage, red cabbage—Shred finely.

Carrots, celery root, beets, white radishes, salsify, kohlrabi—Grate finely or coarsely.

Cucumber, zucchini, radishes, cauliflower—Cut in very thin slices.

Dressings for Raw Vegetables*

29. Oil Dressing*

1 tbsp. oil
1 tsp. lemon juice
1 tsp. fresh herbs or 1 pinch dried herbs

Mix all ingredients well.

30. Mayonnaise

For 6-8 servings:

1 egg yolk, beaten
20 tbsp. oil
A few drops of lemon juice

Add the oil slowly, drop by drop, to the egg yolk, stirring evenly with the whisk.

For 1 serving:

1 tbsp. mayonnaise
1 tsp. lemon juice
1 tsp. fresh herbs or 1 pinch dried herbs

Mix all ingredients well.

31. Mayonnaise with Soy Flour

Vegetable diet when animal protein is forbidden; soy flour replaces egg.

2 level tbsp. soybean flour
6 tbsp. water
15 tbsp. oil
3 tbsp. lemon juice

Blend flour and water to a smooth paste. Alternately, add oil and lemon juice, while constantly and slowly stirring with a whisk.

For 1 serving:

The same as for Mayonnaise, recipe No. 30.

*Use different kinds, depending on doctor's prescription.

32. Cream Dressing

2 tbsp. cream
1 tsp. cottage cheese
1 tsp. lemon juice
1 tsp. fresh herbs or 1 pinch dried herbs

Mix all ingredients well with a whisk.

33. Yogurt Dressing

Low-fat diet

2-3 tbsp. yogurt
A few drops lemon juice
1 tsp. fresh or 1 pinch dried herbs

Mix all ingredients well with a whisk.

34. Almond Puree Dressing

Diet without animal protein

1 tbsp. almond puree
3 tbsp. water
1 tsp. lemon juice
1 tsp. fresh or 1 pinch dried herbs

Slowly add water to almond puree, stirring until creamy. Add lemon juice and herbs.

Salads

For cleaning and reducing the size of raw vegetables, see pages 55-57. Add finely chopped onion or onion juice only in Diets IV and V. Fresh parsley can be added to any salad.

35. Boston Lettuce

Leave whole and use oil dressing.

36. Loose-Leaved Lettuce

Leave whole and use oil dressing.

37. Endive

Cut into strips 1/2 in. wide and use oil dressing or mayonnaise and parsley.

38. Romaine Lettuce

Cut into strips 1/2 in. wide and use oil dressing or mayonnaise, basil, marjoram.

39. Leaf—Bowl Lettuce

Leave whole and use oil dressing or mayonnaise.

40. Cress

Leave whole and use oil dressing or mayonnaise.

41. Spinach

Cut into strips 1/2 in. wide and use oil dressing or mayonnaise, peppermint.

42. Cabbages (only for Diets IV, V): white cabbage, sauerkraut, Brussels sprouts, Savoy cabbage, Chinese cabbage

Shred and toss with oil dressing or mayonnaise, lovage, savory, thyme, caraway seed.

43. Tomatoes

Slice or dice and top with oil dressing or mayonnaise.

44. Fennel

Slice thinly with a knife then chop and add oil dressing or mayonnaise, basil, thyme, dill.

45. Bell Pepper

Cut into thin strips and add oil dressing or mayonnaise.

46. White Radish

Slice or grate and toss with oil dressing or cream dressing.

47. Radish

Slice and add oil dressing or cream dressing.

48. Celery Stalks

Slice thin. Add oil dressing or cream dressing.

49. Zucchini

Slice or grate coarsely. Add oil dressing or mayonnaise, dill, borage, basil.

50. Carrots

Grate thin with cream dressing or oil dressing, marjoram, lovage.

51. Celery Root

Grate thin and top with cream dressing or oil dressing, basil, thyme.

52. Beets

Grate thin or coarse and add cream dressing or mayonnaise, lovage, thyme, caraway.

53. Cauliflower

Cut off flowers, grate stalks. Top with cream dressing or mayonnaise, basil, marjoram, walnuts.

54. Belgian Endive

Cut in 1/2 in. strips. Add cream dressing or oil dressing, tarragon, marjoram.

55. Jerusalem Artichoke

Grate and add cream dressing, thyme.

56. Kohlrabi

Slice and chop or grate with chopping knife and mix with cream dressing or oil dressing, thyme, lovage.

57. Red Cabbage

Slice or mince and add cream dressing or oil dressing, some grated apple, caraway seed, lovage.

58. Mixed Raw Vegetables

Belgian endive with diced tomatoes (oil or mayonnaise dressing)

Bell pepper and fennel (oil dressing)

Fennel, Belgian endive, and diced tomatoes (mayonnaise)

Fennel and carrots (cream dressing)

Cauliflower and carrots (cream dressing)

Tomatoes and bell pepper (oil or mayonnaise dressing)

59. Raw Tomatoes, Stuffed with:

Cucumbers (oil or mayonnaise dressing)

Celery root (cream dressing)

Cauliflower (cream dressing)

60. Sprouted Cereal Grains

Wheat, rye, oats, barley (whole grains)

1st day,
evening: Wash grains in colander under running water,

place in a small bowl and cover with water. Let stand at room temperature.

2nd day,
morning: Rinse and spread out to dry on a plate at room temperature.

evening: Place in a small bowl and cover again with water. Let stand at room temperature.

3rd day,
morning: Rinse and spread out on a plate to dry.

evening: Place in a small bowl and cover with water. Let stand at room temperature.

The grains should have developed sprouts 1/2–3/4 in. long.

61. Special Child's Cereal

Soak cracked grains (groats), mix in blender with bananas, honey, and water.

Sauerkraut

An especially valuable raw vegetable, particularly in winter. It is more easily digestible raw than cooked. Low-salt dietetic sauerkraut is recommended as a raw food. Taste and digestibility of cooked sauerkraut can be improved by adding shredded fresh sauerkraut. Highly recommended for a hypoacid stomach and sluggish intestine: Chew a small amount, once daily.

62. Sauerkraut Salad

Sauerkraut
3-4 crushed juniper berries
few caraway seeds
1 apple
few drops lemon juice
2 tbsp. olive oil

Chop sauerkraut, add caraway seeds (or even crushed

caraway), crushed juniper berries, apple cut in fine strips, lemon juice and olive oil. Any raw tuberous vegetable makes a fine addition.

Pureed Raw Vegetables

If the doctor prescribes pureed food, certain raw vegetables can be mixed in a blender together with the dressing. This makes a good transition from a raw vegetable diet in juice form to a normal raw food diet.
Examples of Blends:

1. 1 small tomato (2-1/2 oz.), handful of spinach (1 oz.), 1 medium carrot (2-1/2 oz.), 1 tsp. onions (if permitted), 1 pinch marjoram.
   Oil dressing: 2 tbsp. sunflower seed oil, 1 tbsp. lemon juice.

2. 1 small tomato (2-1/2 oz.), handful of Boston lettuce (1 oz.), 1 small piece of celery root (1 oz.).
   Cream dressing: 1-2 tbsp. cream, a few drops lemon juice and some lovage.

3. Beets (1 oz.), zucchini (1-1/2 oz.), handful of Boston lettuce (1 oz.).
   Cream dressing: 1/2 oz. cream cheese, 2 tbsp. cream, 1 tbsp. yogurt, possibly some dill; onion if permitted.

4. Celery root (1-1/2 oz.), 1 small carrot (1-1/2 oz.), handful of spinach (1/2 oz.).
   Almond puree dressing: 1 tbsp. almond puree, 1 tbsp. lemon juice, 4 tbsp. water, some rosemary, some minced onion, if permitted.

VI.
Recipes for Cooked Foods

Butter, Vegetable Fats, Oils*

Gastrointestinal patients must be especially careful in using fats.

Health food store vegetable margarine and cooking fats	Vegetable fat emulsions of natural solid fats like cocoa oil or palm seed oil in combination with as high an amount as possible of liquid oils and seed oils, particularly sunflower seed oil
Fresh butter	Use very sparingly
Cold-pressed sunflower seed oil	Used in salad dressings
Linseed oil Poppy seed oil Olive oil	These oils are rich in highly unsaturated fatty acids, also very valuable as a cooking fat because of their purity, and more easily digestible than clarified for cooking vegetables. Never overheat.

Soups

In our soup and vegetable recipes, we use quite a lot of vegetable broth. Since in a small household fresh vegetable broth cannot be prepared daily, water with liquid health food store yeast extract or vegetable bouillon cubes can be used in-

*Unless otherwise specified, use only health food store vegetable fats in the following recipes.

stead. Cream improves the taste of any soup or vegetable, but milk can also be used in place of cream.

Health food store yeast extracts are yeast products rich in vitamin B (glutathione and lecithin).

63. Vegetable Broth

The first recipe is for 4 servings, all others for 1 serving.

Choose vegetables in season, for example, celery root, carrots, some cabbage or kohlrabi, leeks, tomatoes, and onions. Hard but healthy vegetable parts can also be used, as well as potato peelings, etc.

1 tbsp. vegetable fat
1 onion
2 small carrots
1 small celery root (5-1/2 oz.)
Cabbage, mangold leaves
1 leek
3-4 qt. cold water
Lovage and other fresh or dried herbs
1/2 bay leaf
1 pinch salt

Cut unpeeled onion in half and sauté cut surfaces until golden. Cut up vegetables, add to onion and steam, covered, over low heat for at least 1/4 hr. Add the water and simmer for 2 hrs. over low heat, season mildly. Strain and serve as clear broth.

Omit onion if necessary. If this recipe is prepared without fat, add water immediately and simmer very gently for 2 hours.

64. Vegetable Bouillon

1-1/4 cup vegetable broth
health food store yeast extract (opt.)
1/2 oz. fresh butter

Heat broth as prepared in recipe No. 63, and serve with butter and herbs. Season with parsley and chives.

65. Semolina Balls

1/2 oz. butter
1-1/2 tbsp. fine semolina
1/2-1 egg
1 pinch salt
vegetable broth

Cream butter and mix well with semolina. Let stand 1/2 hr. Scoop out small balls with a demitasse spoon, drop in the hot vegetable broth, and simmer gently for 15-20 min. Season with marjoram and nutmeg.

66. Sago Soup and Vegetables

1/2 oz. sago
1/2 qt. vegetable broth
1/2 tbsp. vegetable fat
1 small carrot, diced finely
1 small celery root, diced finely
1 small leek, cut in thin strips
pinch salt

Stir sago into boiling vegetable broth. Sauté vegetables in butter until soft. Add to vegetable broth and simmer for 1/2 hr. Season with health food store yeast extract, parsley, chives.

67. Clear Rice Soup

1/2 tbsp. vegetable fat
Small carrot, thinly sliced
Some celery root, thinly sliced
leek, thinly sliced
1/2 qt. vegetable broth
1 tbsp. rice
pinch salt

Sauté vegetables and rice in fat. Add broth, salt, and simmer 15-20 min.

68. Thick Rice Soup

1/2 tbsp. vegetable fat
Celery, thinly sliced
Small carrot, thinly sliced
Leek, thinly sliced
1 tbsp. rice
1/2 tbsp. flour
2-1/2 cups vegetable broth or water
1/2 tbsp. cream
Chives

Sauté vegetables and rice in fat. Sprinkle with flour and stir. Add liquid and cook 30 min. Serve with cream and chives. Season with 1 pinch salt, health food store yeast extract, parsley, marjoram.

69. Cream of Rice Soup

1 tbsp. rice flour
1/4 tbsp. flour
4 tbsp. milk
2-1/2 cups vegetable broth
1/2 tbsp. butter
1 tbsp. cream

Make a smooth paste of flour and milk and add to the boiling vegetable broth. Cook 1/2 hour. Place in a small soup bowl, with butter and cream. Season with 1 pinch salt, marjoram, possibly nutmeg or caraway seed.

70. Herb Soup

1 tbsp. flour
8 tbsp. milk
1/2 qt. vegetable broth
1 tbsp. cream
1/5 oz. butter or 1 egg yolk, beaten (opt.)

Blend the flour with the cold milk and stir into the boiling vegetable broth. Simmer 15 min. Place cream and butter or egg yolk in a small soup bowl and add the boiling soup to it.

Season with 1 pinch salt, lovage, marjoram, chives, nutmeg or caraway seed.

71. Soybean Soup

1/2 tbsp. vegetable fat
Some onion
1 tbsp. flour
1/2 tbsp. soybean flour
1/2 peeled, diced tomato
1/2 qt. vegetable broth

Sauté onion in vegetable fat. Stir in flours and then add tomatoes and vegetable broth. Season with 1 pinch salt, rosemary, chives, parsley.

72. Cream of Oats Soup

1/2 tbsp. vegetable fat
1/2 tbsp. flour
2 tbsp. rolled oats
2-1/2 cups vegetable broth
Some celery root
1 tbsp. cream

Sauté flour and oats lightly in vegetable fat. Add vegetable broth and celery root. Cook 1 hour and strain. Serve with cream. Season with 1 pinch salt, health food store yeast extract, chives, and possibly nutmeg or caraway seed.

73. Oat Grits Soup

1/2 tbsp. vegetable fat
2 tbsp. oat grits
Some chopped onion
3 cups water or vegetable broth
8 tbsp. milk
Some celery root
Health food store yeast extract
1 tbsp. cream (opt.)

Sauté oat grits and onion in vegetable fat. Add water, milk, and celery root and simmer 1 hour. Serve with yeast extract and cream. Season with 1 pinch salt, chives.

74. Green Rye Soup

1/2 tbsp. vegetable fat
1 tbsp. minced leek
Small cubes of celery root
1-2 tbsp. green rye (whole or coarsely ground), soaked for 12 hrs.
8 tbsp. water
1/2 qt. vegetable broth

Sauté vegetables in fat. Add green rye and steam for a few minutes in 8 tbsp. water. Add vegetable broth and simmer 1–1-1/2 hours. Season with 1 pinch salt, fresh lovage (possibly celery leaves), minced. If necessary, strain or blend soup in a blender.

75. Semolina Soup

1 tbsp. semolina
1/2 qt. vegetable broth
1 egg yolk
1 tbsp. cream
1 pinch salt
nutmeg

Stir semolina into the boiling vegetable broth and simmer 15 minutes. Beat egg yolk, cream, salt and nutmeg together. Add to the boiling soup and serve immediately. Season with health food store yeast extract, minced caraway seed, possibly nutmeg, 1 clove, or chives.

76. Tomato Soup, I

1/2 tbsp. vegetable fat
Some onion
2 tbsp. small carrots
Herb bouquet of minced celery root, leek, garlic clove, some rosemary
1 tomato
1 tbsp. flour
3/5 qt. vegetable broth
Some tomato paste (opt.)
1 tsp. butter
1 tbsp. cream

Add tomato and stir in flour. Add vegetable broth, simmer 1/2 hr. and strain. Serve with butter and cream. Season with 1 pinch salt, cloves, chives, or a bay leaf. Note: 1 tbsp. rice or sago can be used as a filler.

77. Tomato Soup, II

4 ripe tomatoes
1 tsp. lemon juice or 1 tsp. sugar (opt.)
2 tbsp. cream

Cut tomatoes into pieces, boil for a few minutes and strain. Add cream and serve the soup lukewarm or cold.

78. Carrot Soup

1/2 tbsp. vegetable fat
Some onions
1 chopped carrot
1-1/2 tbsp. flour
1/2 qt. vegetable broth
8 tbsp. milk
1 tsp. caraway seed
Celery salt or lovage
1 tbsp. cream

Sauté onions and carrots in the vegetable oil. Stir in flour and sauté. Add vegetable broth, milk, caraway seed, and celery salt. Simmer for 1/2 hr., and then strain. Serve with cream and season with rosemary or marjoram.

79. Spinach Soup (Diets IV, V only)

(Do not eat if you have diarrhea)

1/2 tbsp. vegetable fat
1/2 clove of garlic
1-1/2 tbsp. flour
1/2 qt. vegetable broth
8 tbsp. milk
1 small cup spinach
A few peppermint leaves
1 tbsp. cream
Nutmeg

Sauté garlic and flour in fat. Add vegetable broth and simmer 20 minutes. Mince spinach and peppermint leaves and mix with milk. Add to the finished soup. Serve immediately with cream and nutmeg. Season with 1 pinch salt, parsley, chives, health food store yeast extract, possibly sage.

80. Chervil Soup

1/2 tbsp. vegetable fat
Some onions
1 average size potato, diced
1/2 tbsp. flour
1/2 qt. vegetable broth
1 tbsp. chopped chervil
1 tbsp. cream
1 pinch salt

Sauté onions, potato, and flour in fat. Add vegetable broth, simmer 1/2 hr. and strain. Add cream, chervil and salt and serve.

81. Spring Soup

1/2 tbsp. vegetable fat
1 tbsp. flour
1/2 qt. water or vegetable broth
Some onion
1 tbsp. tender carrots
Spinach leaves*
8 tbsp. milk
1 tbsp. cream

Brown flour in vegetable oil. Add vegetable broth and simmer 1/2 hr. Mince vegetables and add to soup. Allow to stand (covered) a few minutes. Add milk. Place cream in a small soup tureen, add soup and serve. Season with 1 pinch salt, lovage, sorrel, stinging nettle, or dandelion leaves.

82. Cream of Leek Soup

1/2 tbsp. vegetable fat
1/4 leek, coarsely cut
1-1/2 tbsp. flour
3/5 qt. vegetable broth
1 tbsp. cream
1 egg yolk (opt.)

Sauté leek in fat until the leek falls apart and add flour. Add vegetable broth, simmer 1/2–3/4 hr., and strain. Place cream in a small soup tureen and serve. Season with health food store yeast extract, nutmeg, and egg yolk if desired.

83. Potato and Leek Soup

1/2 tbsp. vegetable fat
1/2 leek, cut into thin strips
1/2 tbsp. flour
1/2 qt. vegetable broth
1 med. sized potato, diced
1 tbsp. cream

Sauté leek in fat and stir in flour. Add vegetable broth and

*If no tendency to diarrhea exists.

potato and simmer gently for 10 min. Place cream in a small soup tureen, add soup and serve. Season with 1 pinch salt, health food store yeast extract, and marjoram.

84. Minestra

1/2 tbsp. vegetable fat
Some onion
2 tbsp. leek
A few celery leaves
Handful Romaine lettuce leaves
2-1/2 cups water or vegetable broth
1 tbsp. lovage or thyme
1/2 garlic clove
1/2 oz. whole wheat noodles or brown rice
1/5 oz. butter

Sauté onion in vegetable oil. Mince vegetables and sauté with onions slowly. Add water, seasonings and simmer 1/2 hr. Add noodles after 10 min. so that they cook for 15-20 min. Add butter to improve flavor and season with 1 pinch salt, parsley, and chives.

Vegetables

85. Chopped Spinach (Diets IV, V)

(Do not eat if you have diarrhea)

Select spinach, remove thick stems and wash thoroughly.

7 oz. spinach
1/2 tbsp. vegetable fat
Some garlic
1 tbsp. flour
Spinach water
1 pinch salt
1 cup raw spinach

Dip spinach in boiling water for a second, chop, or blend. Sauté flour and garlic in oil. Add vegetable broth, water, and salt and simmer for 15 min. Add spinach and heat very briefly. Chop raw spinach very fine or blend and add to soup before serving. Season with peppermint leaves, sage, and fresh butter.

86. Romaine Lettuce

1 head Romaine lettuce
1 qt. water
1/2 tbsp. vegetable fat
8 tbsp. vegetable broth
2 tbsp. cream
1 pinch salt

Cut lettuce in half, boil in water until medium soft, and place in a heat-resistant dish. Heat fat slightly and pour over lettuce. Add vegetable broth and salt and bake in 350° oven for 30-40 min. Pour cream over dish 5 minutes before serving.

87. Endive

1 large head endive lettuce

Prepare like Romaine lettuce in recipe No. 86.

88. Belgian Endive

2 cleaned heads Belgian Endive
1/2 tbsp. vegetable fat
2 tbsp. milk or cream
1 tbsp. vegetable broth
Some fresh butter
1 pinch salt

Cut crosswise (1/2 in.) into the stalk. Melt fat and place the Belgian Endive in it. Add cream and vegetable broth and steam (covered) for 1/2 hr. over low heat. Add butter, season and serve. Season with marjoram.

88a. Swiss Chard or Mock Asparagus (Do not eat when flatulent)

3-4 pieces Swiss chard, cleaned
1/2 tbsp. vegetable fat

1/2 small chopped onion
2 tbsp. milk or a little lemon juice
8 tbsp. vegetable broth

Cut Swiss chard into 3-in. long pieces and place in a pan. Sauté onion in oil and pour over stalks. Add milk and vegetable broth and simmer gently over low heat for 1/2–3/4 hr. Season with tarragon, parsley, and chives, and serve the Swiss chard on a platter. Rémoulade sauce can be served with it (allowed in advanced convalescence).

Note: The vegetables can also be served with grated cheese and fresh butter sprinkled over them.

89. Celery Stalks

3-4 peeled celery stalks
1/2 tbsp. vegetable fat
1/2 chopped onion
8 tbsp. vegetable broth
2 tbsp. milk or a little lemon juice
1 pinch salt

Cut celery into pieces 3-1/2 in. long and place in a pan. Sauté with onion in the vegetable fat. Add vegetable broth, milk and salt and simmer gently 1/2–3/4 hr. Season with chopped celery leaves and health food store yeast extract.

90. Fennel

1 rather large or 2 small fennel
1/2 tbsp. vegetable fat
A little onion
8 tbsp. vegetable broth
2 tbsp. milk or lemon juice
1/2 tbsp. flour
2-3 tbsp. cream
1 pinch salt

Cut fennel in half and place in a pan. Sauté onion in vegetable fat and pour over fennel. Add vegetable broth and milk and simmer gently. Bring to a boil and pour the flour, cream, and salt over the finished dish.

91. Steamed Carrots

1/2 tbsp. vegetable fat
1/2 small onion
3-4 small carrots sliced (or cut lengthwise)
8 tbsp. vegetable broth

Sauté onion in vegetable fat. Add carrots and vegetable broth and cook gently 1/2–3/4 hr. Season with marjoram and rosemary.

92. Carrots in Sauce, I

1/4 tbsp. vegetable fat
3-4 carrots cut in small slices
1/2 tbsp. oil
1/2 tbsp. flour
4 tbsp. milk
4 tbsp. water or vegetable broth

Sauté carrots in fat until partially soft. Prepare a thin sauce with the oil, flour, milk and vegetable broth. Add the carrots and simmer for about 1/2 hr. until done. Season with onions, parsley, rosemary, and marjoram.

93. Carrots in Sauce, II

3/4 cup vegetable broth
3-4 carrots, cut lengthwise in thin stalks

Béchamel Sauce, recipe No. 158:
 1/4 tbsp. vegetable fat
 1/4 tbsp. fresh butter
 1 level tbsp. flour
 8 tbsp. milk and carrot juice, mixed
1 tbsp. cream
1 pinch salt

Simmer carrots gently in vegetable broth. Prepare Béchamel Sauce. Add cream and salt. Mix the sauce with the cooked carrots and serve. Season with onions, parsley, rosemary, and marjoram.

94. Peas and Carrots

(As soon as peas are allowed, but avoid in cases of meteorism)

Peas:
1/4 tbsp. vegetable fat
A little onion
4 oz. shelled peas
8 tbsp. vegetable broth

Carrots:
1/4 tbsp. vegetable fat
A little onion
5-1/2 oz. peeled carrots
8 tbsp. vegetable broth
1 pinch salt

Sauté onion and peas in vegetable fat, and simmer in broth until soft. Cut carrots lengthwise into thin stalks, sauté with onion in fat. Add broth and simmer gently until soft. Mix peas and carrots before serving, or serve separately. Season with parsley, chives, and marjoram.

95. Peas

1/2 tbsp. vegetable fat
Some onion
1/2 tbsp. sugar
1/2 lb. shelled peas
8 tbsp. vegetable broth
1 pinch salt
1/2 oz. melted butter

Sauté onion in vegetable fat with sugar. Steam peas in vegetable broth, salt and butter over very low heat until peas are soft (20-40 min.), depending on quality. Pour butter over peas. Season with chives, marjoram, and thyme.

96. French Peas

1/2 tbsp. vegetable fat
1/2 onion
1/4 head lettuce or Romaine lettuce, shredded
5-1/2–7 oz. shelled peas
8 tbsp. vegetable broth
1 pinch salt
1/2 oz. fresh butter, 1 tsp. flour

Sauté onion in vegetable fat. Add lettuce to onion and sauté. Add peas, vegetable broth, and salt, and cook over very low heat until tender. At the last add butter and flour mitxure. Season with chives and marjoram.

97. Steamed Chinese Peas (Diets IV, V)

1/2 tbsp. vegetable fat
1/2 chopped onion
7 oz. cleaned Chinese peas
8 tbsp. vegetable broth
Some parsley or lovage
1 pinch salt

Sauté onion in vegetable fat. Add peas and vegetable broth and steam for 1/2–1 hr., tightly covered. Steam lovage and salt with other ingredients or sprinkle over peas before serving. Season with chives, marjoram and thyme. Melt fresh butter over dish.

97a. Green Beans (Diets IV, V)

(Avoid in cases of meteorism)

1/2 tbsp. vegetable fat
1/2 chopped onion
A little garlic
1/2 lb. green beans
Savory, parsley
1-2 finely diced tomatoes
1 pinch salt

Sauté onion and garlic in vegetable fat. Add beans and parsley and sauté. Add tomatoes (instead of vegetable broth) and simmer over very low heat until beans are soft (about 1 hr.). Add a little broth if necessary. Season with summer savory.

97b. Steamed Celery Root

1/2 tbsp. vegetable fat
1/2 onion
1/2 celery root, peeled and quartered
8 tbsp. vegetable broth
1 tbsp. cream
1 pinch salt

Sauté onion in fat. Slice celery root and sauté. Add vegetable broth and cook gently 1/2–3/4 hr. Add cream and salt to improve flavor. Season with lemon and marjoram.

98. Creamed Celery Root

1 average sized celery root, quartered
4 tbsp. milk
1/2 qt. water
1 pinch salt
Béchamel Sauce, recipe No. 159

Steam celery root in milk, water and salt until done. Cut into slices 1/3 in. thick and arrange on a hot platter with slices overlapping. Serve with Béchamel Sauce.

99. Steamed Salsify (Diet V)

(Avoid in cases of meteorism)

9 oz. cleaned salsify
1/2 tbsp. vegetable fat
1/2 onion
4 tbsp. milk
8 tbsp. vegetable broth
1 pinch salt

Cut salsify into finger-length pieces and place in a pan. Sauté onion slightly in vegetable fat and add to salsify. Add milk, vegetable broth, and salt and cook 1 hr. over low heat. Season with lemon, basil, chopped celery leaves and health food store yeast extract.

100. Beets

12 1/2 oz. beets
1/2 tbsp. vegetable fat
1/2 onion
8 tbsp. vegetable broth
1 pinch sugar
1/4 bay leaf
1/2 tbsp. flour, blended into a paste with cold water
1 tbsp. cream
1 pinch salt

Cut off beet root tips and leaves about 1 in., wash well, without damaging the skin. Cook beets in water gently 2-3 hr., or 25 min. in a pressure cooker. Peel and cut into thin slices. Sauté onion in vegetable fat and add to beets. Add vegetable broth, sugar and bay leaf, mix all ingredients well, and cook gently 1/4 hr. For thickening add flour paste, salt. Serve with cream. Season with lemon, lovage, caraway seed, lemon balm, nutmeg, very little garlic, and parsley.

101. Jerusalem Artichoke

9 oz. Jerusalem artichoke
1/2 tbsp. vegetable fat
1/2 onion
1 tbsp. cream
1 pinch salt

Prepare artichoke like potatoes in their jackets, recipe No. 123. Peel and slice. Sauté onion in fat and add the artichoke, to heat. Add cream and salt to improve flavor. Season with basil.

102. Tomatoes

4-5 tomatoes
1 tbsp. oil

1/2 tbsp. vegetable fat
1/2 onion
Pinch of sugar
A little garlic
1 tbsp. cornstarch (opt.)

Dip tomatoes into boiling water for a few minutes and peel. (Very ripe tomatoes can be peeled without blanching.) Sauté onion in oil, fat, and sugar in frying pan. Quarter tomatoes, add to onions and cook until they are almost done. Add garlic and finish cooking. Add cornstarch to thicken. Sprinkle a little chopped parsley or other herbs such as rosemary, marjoram, basil, and chives over the prepared tomatoes.

103. Steamed Tomatoes

2-3 tomatoes
1/2 oz. butter
1 pinch salt

Cut tomatoes in half and place on a greased cookie sheet or in a baking dish. Place a dab of butter and some salt on each half and bake about 15 min. in a 350 degree oven.

Note: If desired, a few tomatoes can be placed in a blender or finely minced, mixed with cream, brought to a quick boil, and poured over the prepared tomatoes. Season with parsley and onions, sauteéd and sprinkled over tomatoes.

104. Stuffed Tomatoes

2-3 tomatoes
3 tsp. rice (1 tsp. per tomato)
1 pinch salt
Butter
Herbs
Vegetable broth (opt.)

Cut tops off tomatoes (save) and hollow out, chop up tomato pulp, mix with rice and season to taste with herbs. Stuff tomatoes with mixture, put a dab of butter on top, and cover with the cut tops. Bake for 30 min. at 350 degrees. If preferred, sprinkle with some grated cheese. Season with onions, garlic, rosemary and basil.

105. Tomatoes with Scrambled Egg

1-2 tomatoes
1 large egg
1 tbsp. cream
1 pinch salt

Prepare tomatoes like steamed tomatoes, recipe No. 103. Beat egg, cream, and salt together with a whisk. Season with chives.

106. Zucchini

1/2 tbsp. vegetable fat
Chopped onion
1 tbsp. oil
10-1/2 oz. zucchini
2 oz. tomatoes
1 small chopped onion
1 pinch salt

Sauté onion in vegetable fat. Dice zucchini. (If overgrown, remove the inner core.) Peel tomatoes and dice. Steam tomatoes with onion and add last to the prepared zucchini or cook the raw diced tomato with the zucchini. Sprinkle with salt. If too much liquid has formed, add some cornstarch and a little water. Season with garlic, rosemary, marjoram, basil and dill.

107. Peperonata

(With hypoacid, but not hyperacid, stomach)

2 oz. bell pepper
4 oz. zucchini
2 oz. eggplant
1 tomato
1/2 onion
A little garlic
1 tbsp. oil

2 oz. potatoes
1 pinch salt

Cut vegetables in half, remove seeds, and dice. Peel tomato and cut into large cubes. Mince onion in oil and garlic, sauté, and cook with vegetables. Cut potatoes into 1/2-in. cubes, mix and cook all ingredients 1–1-1/2 hrs. If too much juice forms, remove lid and steam. Season with rosemary, marjoram, and thyme.

108. Eggplant, I

14-18 oz. diced eggplant
1-1/2 tbsp. vegetable fat
1 small chopped onion
Vegetable broth (opt.)
Salt to taste

Wash and (if desired) peel eggplant. Sauté onion in vegetable fat. Simmer eggplant with broth and onion until tender. Sprinkle with salt. Garnish with Steamed Tomatoes (recipe No. 103) or with fresh ones.

109. Steamed Cabbage* or White Cabbage (Diet V)

(Avoid with meteorism, but raw cabbage juice is always permitted.) Chew all cabbage well.

1/2 tbsp. vegetable fat
1/2 chopped onion
9 oz. young cabbage
8 tbsp. vegetable broth
Basil or lovage
Health food store yeast extract (opt.)
Nutmeg, caraway seed and 1 pinch salt (opt.)

Sauté onion in oil. Cut cabbage into 1-inch strips, add onion and steam until the vegetable falls apart. Add vegetable

*As a matter of course, doctors seem to forbid cabbage for a gastrointestinal diet. Organically grown cabbage, however, is a valuable vegetable rich in vitamins K and U. As juice or pureed in blender, it is easily digestible in all conditions; cooked whole, it is also safe for the convalescent (Diet V). Try in small amounts first, salivate and chew well.

broth and simmer gently for 1/2 hr. over low heat. Season with herbs and serve with some garlic and parsley.

Note: Grown out cabbage must first be dipped briefly in boiling water.

110. Chopped Cabbage (Diet V)

7 oz. cabbage
1 qt. water
1/2 tbsp. vegetable fat
1/2 chopped onion
Some garlic
1 small tbsp. flour
8 tbsp. vegetable broth or 4 tbsp. milk and 4 tbsp. vegetable broth
1-2 tbsp. cream
Health food store yeast extract
Nutmeg
1 pinch salt

Cut cabbage into 4 pieces, cook gently in water and drain, chop finely. Sauté onion in vegetable fat. Sprinkle garlic over. Add flour and broth and simmer 15 min. Add cabbage and cook slightly. Add cream and season to taste. Season with caraway seed and parsley.

111. Red Cabbage (Diet V)

(Avoid in cases of meteorism)

1/2 tbsp. vegetable fat
1/2 chopped onion
9 oz. thin sliced red cabbage
1/2 tbsp. lemon juice
1/2 apple, sliced thin
1/2 tbsp. rice
8 tbsp. vegetable broth
4 tbsp. grape juice or apple juice
1 peeled apple, sliced
Some butter
1 pinch salt

Sauté onion in vegetable fat. Add cabbage, lemon juice,

apple, and rice and sauté together. Pour broth and fruit juice over mixture and simmer covered over low heat for 1–1-1/2 hrs. Brush apple with butter and bake on a cookie sheet. Salt cabbage dish and garnish with baked apple slices.

112. Kohlrabi with Herbs (Diet IV, V)

(Avoid at first in cases of meteorism)

1 kohlrabi
1/2 tbsp. vegetable fat
1/2 chopped onion
8 tbsp. vegetable broth
1 tbsp. tender kohlrabi leaves, chopped
1 tbsp. cream
1 pinch salt
Béchamel Sauce (recipe No. 158)

Cut kohlrabi into thin slices. Heat fat and add vegetables. Add onion and broth and cook covered 1/2–1 hr. Add kohlrabi leaves, cream, and sprinkle with salt. Mix various other chopped herbs with Béchamel Sauce and add to cooked kohlrabi.

113. Leek (Diet II)

(Avoid in cases of meteorism)

7 oz. cleaned leeks
1/2 tbsp. vegetable fat
8 tbsp. vegetable broth
1 tbsp. cream
1 pinch salt
Some grated cheese (opt.)

Cut leeks into 3-inch strips. Place vegetable fat and broth in a frying pan and cook slowly, covered. Add cream and sprinkle with salt.

114. Onions

(Avoid in cases of meteorism)

1/2 tbsp. vegetable fat
7 oz. pearl onions
1 pinch sugar
8 tbsp. vegetable broth

Sauté onions in vegetable fat and sugar. Add broth and cook another 3/4 hr. The vegetables can be garnished with peas or with Béchamel Sauce (recipe No. 158).

115. Chestnuts (Diet V only)

9 oz. chestnuts
1/2 tbsp. vegetable fat
1/2 tbsp. sugar
8 tbsp. vegetable broth
1 tbsp. cream
1 pinch salt
Fresh butter

Clean chestnuts, allow to swell in a hot oven, and then peel. Sauté chestnuts in vegetable fat until brown. Mix sugar, salt, broth and cream and add to chestnuts. Season and cook about 1/2 hr. until liquid is absorbed. Place dabs of butter on the prepared chestnuts.

Note: Take small bites at a time and chew thoroughly.

116. Mixed Vegetables

1/2 tbsp. health store vegetable fat
1/2 onion
2 oz. celery root
2 oz. carrots
8 tbsp. vegetable broth
2 oz. cauliflower
8 tbsp. milk and water
2 oz. peas or beans
8 tbsp. vegetable broth
1 pinch salt

Sauté onion in vegetable fat. Cut vegetables into small cubes and sauté with onions. Add broth and cook thoroughly. Cook cauliflower gently in some milk-water. Cook peas gently in broth and salt.

Cooked Vegetable Salads

Carrots, celery root, beets, beans and cauliflower are especially suitable for these salads (beans and cauliflower should not be eaten in cases of meteorism).

The vegetables are cooked gently in vegetable broth or water and then cut up small into cubes, slices, or florets. They are dressed with salad dressings or diluted mayonnaise. Use chopped herbs as seasonings.

117. Potato Salad (Diet V)

7 oz. potatoes, boiled in their skins
4 tbsp. hot vegetable broth
1 tbsp. oil
1 tbsp. lemon juice
1/2 tbsp. cream
1/2 tbsp. chopped onion (if digestible)
1 pinch salt

Peel the hot boiled potatoes and slice. Pour broth over potatoes and let stand. Beat onion, lemon juice, cream and salt well and mix with the potatoes while still warm. Season with borage, sour milk, parsley, lemon balm, and dill.

118. Potato Salad with Cucumbers (If cucumbers are digestible)

1 large potato, prepared as in recipe No. 117
1/4 cucumber
1/2 tbsp. oil
1/2 tbsp. lemon juice
1 pinch salt

Prepare potato as in Potato Salad, recipe No. 117. Grate cucumber on a coarse grater. Mix cucumber with sauce of oil, lemon juice, and salt and potato salad. Serve in a bowl rubbed with garlic. Season with dill and chives.

119. Mixed Salad
(from cooked vegetables)

For example, carrots, celery root, zucchini, beets, and potatoes. For this salad, use 3-4 different cooked vegetables, diced or sliced, and mix them with the salad dressing. Season with health food store yeast extract, chives, parsley and dill.

120. Niçoise Salad

Radishes
1 cooked potato
1 small tomato
1 hard-boiled egg
A few cucumber slices
1 tbsp. oil
1/2 tbsp. lemon juice
A few leaves Boston lettuce
1 pinch salt

Slice vegetables and egg. Mix oil, lemon juice and seasonings and mix with the vegetables and egg. Add lettuce to salad shortly before serving. Season with chives or dill, borage.

121. Rice Salad

2 oz. rice
1 cup water
1 tbsp. oil
1/2 tbsp. lemon juice
1/2 chopped onion
1/2 tomato, in thin cubes

Cook rice in water, rinse, and let cool. Beat oil, lemon juice and onion into a sauce and mix with the rice. Add tomatoes and season with chives, parsley, or basil.

Serve the prepared salad on lettuce leaves, or serve in clam shells for special occasions.

122. Vegetable Aspic

1 cup lukewarm vegetable broth
1/10 oz. powdered agar-agar*
1 pinch salt
A few drops lemon juice
Health food store yeast extract
Fresh cucumbers
Small tomato cubes
Cooked cauliflower tips
Cooked peas
Cooked beans

Dissolve agar-agar in broth and heat slowly until the agar-agar is completely dissolved. Add salt, lemon juice and yeast extract. Place a little jelly in rinsed out molds, then allow to become solid. Garnish with egg and vegetable slices, pour some vegetable broth over, and allow to set, etc., until the mold is filled. Invert the cooled jelly and garnish on a salad platter.

Potato Dishes

123. Potatoes in Their Jackets

3-4 small potatoes (red or yellow potatoes are preferable)
Water
1 pinch salt

Brush off potatoes and wash. Place potatoes in pan with perforated insert or wire basket. Fill water up to insert, add salt, cover and steam 30-40 minutes, or cook in a pressure cooker.

*Agar-agar is a vegetable gelatin, available as a powder and used for vegetable aspics and fruit jellies, sauces, and puddings, etc., instead of animal gelatin. It is especially beneficial for gastric patients, since fruit and vegetable juices and the vegetables "jelled" in the agar-agar are easily digestible and soothing and are therefore very valuable.

124. Baked Potatoes

3-4 small potatoes
1 tbsp. oil
Some salt
Butter

Brush potatoes and wash. Make 3-4 slits in the skin on the top side, brush with oil, and bake at 350 degrees on a greased sheet for 30-40 min. Place a dab of butter on each of the potatoes.

125. Potatoes with Cottage Cheese

3-4 small potatoes
1 tbsp. oil

Filling:
2 oz. cottage cheese
1-2 tbsp. milk or cream
Chives or caraway seed or marjoram
1 pinch salt

Make a slit in the top side of the potatoes and prepare like baked potatoes. Beat cottage cheese and milk until frothy and mix with other ingredients. Season and place filling in the deep ridge of the baked potato. This mixture can also be served with baked potatoes.

126. Caraway Seed Potatoes

2-3 medium-sized potatoes (oblong, slender)
1 tsp. caraway seed
1 pinch salt

Brush potatoes and wash. Cut in half lengthwise. Mix caraway seed and salt and sprinkle on potatoes; place the cut surface face down on a greased sheet, brush with oil and bake for 3/4 hr. at 350 degrees.

127. Bouillon Potatoes

9 oz. potatoes
8-16 tbsp. vegetable broth
1 pinch salt
1/2 oz. butter

Wash potatoes, peel, cut in half or in pieces and cook gently in salted broth. Place dab of butter on potatoes and season with lovage, some thyme, and bay leaf.

128. Parsley Potatoes

9 oz. peeled potatoes
A little water
1 tbsp. fresh butter
1 tbsp. chopped parsley
1 pinch salt

Cut potatoes into 4 pieces, lengthwise. Steam potatoes with water on a perforated insert. Melt butter and pour over potatoes. Sprinkle with parsley and salt and serve.

129. Cream Potatoes

7 oz. potatoes
1/2 tbsp. vegetable fat
8 tbsp. vegetable broth
4 tbsp. cream or milk
Parsley
1 pinch salt

Slice potatoes into small pieces. Sauté slightly in vegetable fat and cook gently with the vegetable broth. Add cream and sprinkle with parsley and salt. Season with thyme, small cloves, nutmeg and health food store yeast extract.

130. Potatoes with Tomatoes

1/2 tbsp. vegetable fat
7 oz. potatoes
8 tbsp. vegetable broth
1 small tomato
1 tbsp. cream
1 pinch salt

Sauté peeled sliced potatoes in oil and cook in vegetable broth until semi-soft. Add peeled, sliced tomato and cook until done. Add cream and salt. Season with marjoram or rosemary or thyme and possibly nutmeg.

131. Mashed Potatoes, I

4 potatoes
water
1 pinch salt

Wash potatoes, peel, and cut into pieces. Steam (with little water) until soft. Press through a potato press onto a warm platter. Pour melted butter over potatoes and sprinkle with minced tomato.

132. Mashed Potatoes, II

4 potatoes
A little water
1/2 oz. butter
8 tbsp. milk
Nutmeg
1 tbsp. cream (opt.)
1 pinch salt

Peel potatoes, cut into pieces, steam in water until soft. Press through the potato press. Warm butter and milk, add potatoes, beat well and season. Serve on a hot platter. Dip a knife in hot water, and decorate puree. Season with marjoram, caraway seed, and tomatoes all finely minced.

133. Potato Balls

4 potatoes
8 tbsp. milk
1/2 oz. butter

Prepare like mashed potatoes (recipe No. 132). Dip a small scoop into melted butter, scoop out balls of mashed potatoes and serve on a hot platter.

1/2 oz. butter
1 pinch salt

Sprinkle with salt and dot with butter. Season with nutmeg.

134. Smothered Potatoes

11 oz. peeled potatoes
A little water
8 tbsp. vegetable broth
1/2 tbsp. vegetable fat
1-2 tbsp. cream
1 pinch salt

Cut potatoes in half and steam in a little water until semi-soft. Place on a heat-resistant platter, face down. Pour broth and melted fat over potatoes and bake at 350 degrees until the vegetable broth is absorbed. Pour cream over potatoes, sprinkle with salt. Bake until the cut surfaces are slightly browned. Season with some nutmeg and thyme. Serve the smothered potatoes face up and sprinkle with chopped parsley.

135. Princess Potatoes

3 potatoes
A little water
1 tbsp. grated cheese or cottage cheese
1/2 tbsp. vegetable fat
8 tbsp. milk
1 egg
2 tbsp. milk
1 tbsp. cream or milk
Butter dabs
1 pinch salt

Steam, peel, and cut potatoes into thick slices. Place in a baking dish with water. Mix cheese with potatoes. Spread melted vegetable fat and milk over potatoes, bake 10 minutes at 350 degrees. Beat egg and milk together and pour over potatoes. Place dabs of butter on mixture, salt, and bake at 350 degrees 10-15 minutes. Season with nutmeg and marjoram.

Grain Dishes

136. Japanese Rice

1/2 tbsp. vegetable fat
3 oz. rice
12-16 tbsp. vegetable bouillon or celery water
1/2 oz. butter
1 pinch salt

Sauté rice in vegetable fat. Add bouillon and an onion stuck with 2 cloves and cook 15 minutes. Rice should be grainy; let cool. Add soft butter and salt to rice and heat while stirring. Place butter patties over finished rice.

137. Risotto

1/2 tbsp. vegetable fat
1 tbsp. chopped onion
3 oz. rice
4/5 cup vegetable broth or water

1/2 oz. fresh butter
1 pinch salt

Sauté rice with the onion and vegetable fat until transparent. Add hot broth and cook 15-20 min. Mix in butter and salt with a fork. Season with fresh herbs to taste (rosemary).

139. Saffron Rice

Prepare like Risotto (recipe No. 137). Dissolve a pinch of saffron powder in some bouillon and add to rice. Season with fresh herbs to taste and rosemary.

140. Rice Creole

1/2 tbsp. vegetable fat
1/2 tbsp. chopped onion
3 oz. rice
4/5 cup water or vegetable broth
1 pinch salt

Sauté rice, onion and vegetable fat until rice is transparent. Add hot broth and salt and cook 15-20 min. Season with health food store yeast extract.

141. Rice Creole with Vegetables

1/2 tbsp. vegetable fat
2 tbsp. vegetables, diced very fine (leek, celery root, carrots)
3 oz. rice
4/5 cup vegetable broth
1 pinch salt

Steam vegetables, fat, and rice together. Add hot broth and salt and cook 15-20 min. Season with freshly minced herbs to taste.

142. Tomato Rice

1/2 tbsp. vegetable fat
1/2 tbsp. chopped onion
A little garlic
3 oz. rice
1 large tomato
8 tbsp. vegetable broth
1/2 oz. fresh butter
1 pinch salt

Sauté vegetables in fat. Sauté rice with vegetables until transparent. Peel tomato and dice, add to mixture. Add broth and cook 15-20 minutes. Mix in butter and salt. Season with rosemary, basil and nutmeg.

143. Risotto with Bell Pepper

1 tbsp. oil
1 tbsp. chopped onion
1/2 bell pepper, cut in strips
2 oz. rice
8 tbsp. vegetable broth
1 pinch salt

Sauté vegetables in oil. Sauté rice with oil and vegetables. Add broth and salt and bake 15 min. in oven or cook gently. Note: If the bell pepper is rather sharp, cut it up in large pieces and soak in cold water for 1 hr. before cooking.

144. Rice with Zucchini

1/2 tbsp. vegetable fat
1 tbsp. chopped onion
5-1/2 oz. tender zucchini
Some vegetable broth or water
3 oz. rice
12 tbsp. water or vegetable broth
1/2 oz. butter
1 pinch salt

Sauté onion in fat. Dice zucchini and sauté with onion for 10 min. Add rice, and gradually add broth until a risotto forms. Add butter and salt. Season with health food store yeast extract and freshly chopped dill.

145. Rice with Peas

1/2 tbsp. vegetable fat
Some chopped onion
Some sugar
5-1/2 oz. shelled peas
4 tbsp. vegetable broth
1/2 tbsp. vegetable fat
Some chopped onion
3 oz. rice
5–6-2/3 oz. water
1/2 oz. butter
1 pinch salt

Sauté onion in vegetable fat and sugar. Add peas and broth and sauté with onion lightly, then simmer gently. Prepare a risotto with fat, onion, rice and water and add the cooked peas last. Top with butter and sprinkle with salt. Season with chopped parsley.

146. Rice with Spinach (Diets IV, V only)

1/2 tbsp. vegetable fat
Some chopped onion
4 oz. coarsely cut spinach
3 oz. rice
4/5 cup vegetable broth or hot water
1/2 oz. fresh butter
1 pinch salt

Sauté onion in vegetable fat. Sauté spinach and rice with onion. Add broth and cook 15-20 minutes. Sprinkle with salt and top with butter. Season with nutmeg and peppermint.

147. Rice Pudding with Tomatoes

1/2 tbsp. vegetable fat
1 tbsp. very finely diced vegetables (leek, celery root, carrots)
3 oz. rice
12 tbsp. vegetable broth
2 small tomatoes, sliced
1/2 oz. butter
1 pinch salt

Sauté vegetables and rice in fat. Add hot broth and cook 15-20 min. Place rice and tomato slices in layers in a buttered baking dish. Place butter patties on top, sprinkle with salt, and bake 10 minutes at 350 degrees. Season with parsley and lovage.

148. Semolina

2 oz. semolina
1-1/4 cup milk
4/5 cup water
1 tbsp. raw sugar
1/2 oz. butter
1 pinch salt

Stir semolina and milk into boiling water and cook 15-20 minutes. Dissolve sugar and salt in butter and pour over prepared semolina. Sprinkle with mixed sugar and cinnamon.

149. Semolina Gnocchi

2 oz. semolina
1-1/4 cup milk
Nutmeg
1 pinch salt

Stir semolina into boiling milk and simmer 15-20 minutes. Spread out on a chopping board, about 1/2 in. thick, sprinkle with nutmeg and salt, and let cool. Cut into small rounds. Place the excess pieces in a buttered heatproof mold and then arrange the rounds over them.

1 egg
4 tbsp. milk
2 tbsp. cream
1 tbsp. chives
1 tbsp. cheese
1/2 oz. butter
1 pinch salt

Beat egg with milk and cream and pour over. Sprinkle with chives, cheese, and salt, and dab with butter. Bake slowly until the mixture has set.

150. Polenta

1/2 tbsp. oil
2 oz. cornmeal
1-1/4 cup water
Nutmeg
1 pinch salt
1 tsp. fresh butter
1 tbsp. grated cheese

Oil pan. Bring water to a boil and add corn, nutmeg, and salt. Simmer 5 minutes over low heat while stirring constantly, then cook 1-2 hrs. over very low heat. Mix in butter and cheese and serve.

151. Millotto

1/2 tbsp. vegetable fat
1/2 tbsp. chopped onion
2 oz. millet
12 tbsp. hot vegetable broth
1 tbsp. cheese, grated
1/2 oz. butter
1 pinch salt

Sauté onion and millet in fat until transparent. Add broth and cook 20 minutes. Sprinkle with salt, butter and cheese before serving.

152. Millotto with Vegetables

1/2 tbsp. vegetable fat
1/2 tbsp. chopped onion
1 tbsp. diced vegetables (leek, celery root, carrots) or carrots and peas
1-1/2 oz. millet
12 tbsp. vegetable broth
1 tbsp. cheese
1/2 oz. butter
1 pinch salt

Sauté millet and vegetables in fat. Add broth and cook 20 minutes. Top with salt, cheese and butter and serve immediately. Season with rosemary and health food store yeast extract.

153. Porridge

2 tbsp. cracked grain (groats) (wheat, oats, rye)
3 tbsp. water
1 pinch salt

Soak grains for 12 hrs. Add 2-3 tbsp. water and salt, cook 20-30 minutes in a double boiler, then blend in a blender if needed.

154. Homemade Noodles

(4 servings)

7 oz. flour (1/2 amt. should be whole wheat)
2 eggs
1-2 tbsp. water
1 tbsp. oil
1 pinch salt

Sift flour onto a pastry board, place remaining ingredients in the center and blend together into a solid dough. Make sure that there are no air holes in dough when cut through. Let stand 1/2 hr. Season with basil and parsley, sautéed lightly in butter and sprinkled over dough.

155. Mini Gnocchi (Diet V)

2-1/2 oz. flour (1/2 of it whole wheat)
1 egg
8 tbsp. milk-water
1 qt. water
1 pinch salt
1 tbsp. cheese
1/2 oz. fresh butter
Chives and parsley

Blend together flour, egg, and milk-water and work dough until it forms bubbles. Let stand at least 1 hr. Bring salted water to a boil. Strain dough partially through a sieve (with large holes) into boiling water and let dumplings simmer until they rise to the surface. Take out with perforated spoon and serve on a hot platter. Sprinkle with cheese, butter and herbs.

When the mini Gnocchi have cooled, they can be placed once more in clear, hot water. Instead of using a sieve, a small amount of dough can be placed on a moist wooden board and thin strips can be cut off and allowed to fall into the boiling water.

156. Soybean Gnocchi (Diet V)

2-1/2 oz. whole wheat flour
1 oz. soybean flour
8 tbsp. water
1 pinch salt

Prepare like recipe No. 155. Season with chives and parsley or tomatoes. The Gnocchi can be cooked in vegetable broth and immediately served on a hot platter.

157. Spinach or Tomato Gnocchi

2-1/2 oz. flour (1/3 whole wheat)
1 egg
8 tbsp. milk-water
1 handful raw, chopped spinach or 1 tsp. tomato paste
1 qt. water
1 pinch salt

Work all ingredients into a smooth dough and let stand 1 hr. Prepare like recipe No. 155, adding spinach to the dough. Season with chives and parsley or tomatoes.

Sauces

158. Béchamel Sauce (Diet V only)

1/2 tbsp. vegetable fat
1/2 tbsp. butter
1 tbsp. flour
4 tbsp. milk
4 tbsp. vegetable broth or water
1 pinch salt

Melt butter and fat, sift in flour and sauté lightly. Add the liquid slowly while stirring vigorously and cook 20 minutes. Season with nutmeg.

159. Herb Sauce

Prepare Béchamel sauce. Thicken with an egg yolk. Season with lovage, chervil, basil, tarragon, etc.

160. Tomato Sauce, I

1 tsp. vegetable fat
1 tbsp. onions
Some garlic
2 tbsp. carrots, celery root, leek
2 small tomatoes
Some flour
12 tbsp. vegetable broth or water
1 pinch salt
Some fresh butter or oil
1 pinch sugar (opt.)

Slice vegetables (except tomatoes) thick and steam all together well in vegetable fat. Cut tomatoes in pieces and sauté with vegetables until the juice is absorbed. Sprinkle flour over, add broth and salt and cook 1/2 hr. Strain. Add butter and sugar to improve taste. Season with rosemary, thyme.

161. Tomato Sauce, II

3 tomatoes
1 tbsp. cream or some fresh butter or oil
1 pinch salt

Cut tomatoes into pieces, steam until soft. Strain. Add cream and salt. Season with chives and basil.

162. Tomato Sauce, III

1/2 tbsp. vegetable fat
1/2 small chopped onion
2 peeled tomatoes

Sauté onion in vegetable fat. Cut tomatoes into cubes and steam until soft. Season with thyme, lemon juice, sugar.

163. Mayonnaise, I (Diets IV, V)

(4 servings)
1 egg yolk
1 tbsp. lemon juice
4/5 cup oil
1 pinch salt

Beat egg yolk well with a few drops of lemon juice. Add the oil drop by drop while stirring evenly with a whisk. If the mayonnaise is too thick, dilute with some lemon juice. Season just before serving with health food store yeast extract and chopped onions and herbs.

164. Mayonnaise, II (4 servings)

1 egg yolk
1 tbsp. lemon juice
8-12 tbsp. oil
8 tbsp. vegetable broth or water
1 level tbsp. flour

Prepare like mayonnaise, recipe No. 163, using first three ingredients. Mix broth and flour until smooth and bring to a boil, let cool. Mix this rather thick sauce slowly with the prepared mayonnaise. Season as in recipe No. 163.

165. Mayonnaise without Animal Protein

(4 servings)

2 level tbsp. soybean flour
6 tbsp. water
4/5 cup oil
4 tbsp. lemon juice

Mix flour and water into a smooth dough. Add oil and lemon juice alternately while stirring constantly with a whisk. Season as in recipe No. 163.

Pastry Doughs and Desserts

166. Shortcrust Pastry

(Recipes serve 4)

7 oz. flour (1/4 whole wheat)
3-4 oz. butter
Salt
4 tbsp. water

Cut butter into flour. Dissolve salt in water, add to flour, and knead lightly until a smooth dough forms. Set aside in a cool place for 1/2 hr.

167. Sweet Shortcrust Pastry (Diet V)

(as an exception)

7 oz. flour
3 oz. butter
1 pinch salt
1 tbsp. raw sugar
1 egg

Cut butter into flour. Add sugar, salt, and egg, and knead lightly until a smooth dough forms. Set aside in a cool place for 1/2 hour.

168. Stewed Fruit

2-4 oz. raw sugar
1-1/2 cups water or 4/5 cup grape juice
28 oz. apricots or peaches, prunes, plums

Add sugar and water and bring to a boil. Remove pits from fruit, cut in half, and cook briefly in syrup. Let cool and serve.

169. Strawberries in Lemon Juice

21 oz. prepared strawberries
1 lemon
2-3 tbsp. raw sugar or honey

Cut large strawberries in half, mix in honey and lemon juice.

170. Fruit Salad with Syrup

4 oz. raw sugar
8 tbsp. water
8-16 tbsp. grape juice or apple juice
1-2 tbsp. lemon juice
21 oz. apricots or peaches
Fresh fruit in season:
- Melons
- Apples
- Pears (soft kinds)
- Pitted red cherries
- All types of berries

Bring sugar and water to a boil and let cool. Add juices and combine with apricots or peaches. Cut fruit into thin slices and place in the prepared syrup.

171. Stuffed Melons

2 small melons
Fruit Salad, recipe No. 170.

Cut melons in half, hollow out and fill with Fruit Salad.

172. Fruit Jelly

1-1/4 cup water or grape juice
3 oz. raw or cane sugar
1/2 oz. powdered agar-agar*
3 cups fruit juice (oranges, berries)

Blend water, sugar, and agar-agar and heat over a low flame, stirring constantly, until the agar-agar has completely dissolved. Mix fruit juice with the agar-agar and serve immediately in glasses or cups. If allowed, garnish with whipped cream to taste.

173. Apple Sauce

28 oz. apples
4/5 cup water or apple juice
3-4 oz. raw sugar
Cinnamon or grated lemon peel

Remove apple cores and stems, cut into pieces, cook in water until soft and strain. Mix sugar and flavoring with apples.

174. Apple Sauce with Meringue Icing (as an exception)

Preparation and ingredients as in recipe No. 173. Serve in a pudding mold. (Serve this dish as an exception.)

2-3 egg whites
4 oz. raw sugar

*See note for recipe No. 122.

Beat egg whites until very stiff, fold in sugar, garnish sauce with meringue squeezed through a pastry bag. Bake briefly at 350 degrees.

175. Apple Compote

28 oz. apples
2–2-1/4 cups water or apple juice
4 oz. cane sugar
Some cinnamon

Peel apples, remove core, and slice. Bring liquid to a boil. Add sugar and cinnamon and boil apples until soft.

176. Apple Halves

28 oz. apples
1/2 qt. water or apple juice
4 oz. cane sugar
1/4 cinnamon stick

Peel apples, cut in halves, hollow out. Bring juice, sugar and flavoring to a boil. Place apples in juice and cook slowly until soft. Remove with a perforated spoon and serve on a flat plate face up. Use quince, raspberry, or currant jelly to stuff apple halves.

177. Blueberry Sauce (slightly constipating)

2 lb. blueberries
4-7 oz. raw sugar
4/5 cup water
1 tbsp. flour
2 tbsp. water
1 oz. butter
1/2 oz. croutons

Clean berries and cook with sugar and water 5-10 minutes. Blend in flour and water and bring to a boil. Brown croutons slightly, top with butter and sauce and serve.

178. Rhubarb Compote
(laxative; only if allowed)

2 lb. rhubarb
5-7 oz. raw sugar
8 tbsp. water
1 tsp. cornstarch (opt.)

Wash rhubarb and dice. Place in pan with sugar and water and boil gently for a few minutes. Remove rhubarb with a perforated spoon and put in a serving dish. Thicken juice with some cornstarch and pour over rhubarb.

179. Strawberry Cup

18 oz. strawberries
4 oz. raw sugar or fruit concentrate
4/5 cup whipping cream

Blend berries or strain through a fine sieve. Add sugar and carefully fold in whipped cream. Garnish with whole berries. Note: Other fruit can also be used in this way.

180. Fruit Cup

9 oz. fruit (pears, apricots, peaches, and berries)
4/5 cup water
2-3 tbsp. raw sugar
Vanilla cream (prepared as in recipe No. 184)
8 tbsp. cream

Boil fruit in water and sugar. Pour vanilla cream over the prepared fruit and garnish with cream.

181. Junket with Fruit

3/4 qt. milk
1-2 tbsp. cane sugar
Vanilla sugar or grated lemon peel

1/2 junket* tablet
1 tbsp. water
Fresh sugared berries
8 tbsp. cream

Warm milk, sugar, and flavoring to about 98.6 degrees F. Dissolve junket in water and add to the warm milk, blend quickly, and pour immediately into glasses. When the junket has set, allow to cool. Sprinkle berries over junket shortly before serving and garnish with whipped cream.

182. Stuffed Apples

4 large or 8 small apples

Filling:

2 tbsp. raisins
4 tbsp. cream
3 tbsp. raw sugar or honey
1 lemon peel, grated

1/2 oz. butter
1 tbsp. raw sugar
8-16 tbsp. apple juice

Remove cores and peel apples. Mix raisins, cream, honey and lemon peel, fill in apples and place in a baking dish. Dab apples with butter and sugar and fill pan with apple juice 1/2 inch deep. Bake 20-30 minutes. Aples can also be baked without filling. If desired serve with some cream.

183. Apple "Hedgehog" with Vanilla Cream

28 oz. apples
1-1/3 cup milk
1/2 vanilla bean
1-2 tbsp. raw or cane sugar
1 tsp. cornstarch
1 egg
8 tbsp. whipping cream
1-1/2 oz. almonds

*See note for recipe No. 22.

Prepare apples as in recipe No. 176. Use next 5 ingredients to prepare Vanilla Cream as in recipe No. 184. Beat cream stiffly and fold in with the Vanilla Cream. Shell almonds, cut into slivers and toast lightly in oven. Serve apples face down on a flat plate, stick almond slivers into apples and top with the vanilla cream.

184. Vanilla Cream

3 cups milk
1 vanilla bean
1 tbsp. cornstarch
3 tbsp. milk
3 eggs
2-4 oz. raw or cane sugar

Bring milk and vanilla to a boil. Remove from heat. Blend cornstarch with milk and add to the hot milk. Lightly beat eggs and sugar and stir in some hot milk. Pour back into the saucepan while stirring well. Do not boil. The cream should have a smooth, heavy flowing texture.

185. Strawberry or Raspberry Cream

11 oz. berries
Cream:
  1 cup milk
  1 tsp. cornstarch
  1 tbsp. milk
  1 egg
  2-3 tbsp. raw sugar

8-16 tbsp. whipping cream

Clean and strain berries. Prepare next 5 ingredients as in Vanilla Cream, recipe No. 184. Allow to cool, and mix with berries. Beat cream stiffly and fold into berries.

186. Apple Cream

Vanilla Cream:

1 cup milk
1/2 vanilla bean
1 tsp. cornstarch
1 tbsp. milk
1 egg
1 tbsp. raw or cane sugar

14 oz. apples
4 tbsp. water or apple juice
2 tbsp. raw or cane sugar
Grated lemon peel
8-16 tbsp. whipping cream

Prepare like Vanilla Cream, recipe No. 184. Prepare a thick apple sauce with apples, apple juice, sugar and lemon peel, and mix with the Vanilla Cream. Beat cream until stiff and fold into apple sauce.

187. Rhubarb Cream

(laxative)

14 oz. rhubarb
4–5-1/2 oz. raw or cane sugar
Vanilla Cream:
1 cup milk
1/2 vanilla bean
1 tsp. cornstarch
1 tbsp. milk
1 egg
1 tbsp. raw sugar or honey
8-16 tbsp. whipping cream

Wash and dice rhubarb. Cook with sugar until tender. Blend or strain. Prepare Vanilla Cream as in recipe No. 184. Let cool and mix with rhubarb. Beat cream stiffly and mix or garnish with the rhubarb cream.

188. Orange Cream

Prepare like Lemon Cream, recipe No. 190, using oranges instead of lemons.

189. Orange Cream (prepared cold)

1 piece orange peel
8 tbsp. water
1 small tsp. powdered agar-agar
4/5 cup orange juice
1 tsp. lemon juice
5-6 tbsp. raw sugar or honey
2 eggs
8-16 tbsp. whipping cream

Beat orange peel, water, agar-agar, and heat slowly over low heat until the powder is well dissolved. Mix juices with the dissolved agar-agar. Stir honey and eggs until frothy and mix in the fruit cream. Beat cream stiffly and fold in carefully. Pour in serving dish and refrigerate 1 hour.

190. Lemon Cream

3 cups milk
Peel of 1-2 lemons
1 tbsp. cornstarch
3 tbsp. milk
3 eggs
3-4 oz. raw or cane sugar
8-16 tbsp. cream

Bring milk and lemon peel to a boil. Remove from heat. Blend cornstarch and milk, add to hot milk, and bring to a boil briefly. Beat eggs and sugar. Add some hot milk, pour back into saucepan while stirring well and heat to below boiling point. Strain the cold cream, add a few tsp. lemon juice and fold in the whipped cream.

191. Lemon Cream (prepared cold)

1 piece lemon peel
12 tbsp. water
1 scant tsp. powdered agar-agar
3-4 tbsp. lemon juice
5-6 tbsp. raw sugar
2 eggs
8-16 tbsp. whipping cream

Prepare like Orange Cream, recipe No. 189.

192. Orange Jelly

1-1/4 cup orange juice
1 small tsp. powdered agar-agar
1 tbsp. raw sugar
4/5 cup orange juice

Blend orange juice, agar-agar and sugar well and heat over a small flame while stirring constantly (do not boil) until the agar-agar is completely dissolved. Add orange juice and dish out in small molds that have been rinsed cold, and chill.

193. Chaudeau

2 eggs
2 oz. raw sugar
12 tbsp. grap juice
1 tbsp. lemon juice

Beat eggs, sugar and juices. Place in a lukewarm double boiler, heat slowly and stir until frothy. Note: If cream is too thick, add a little more grape juice.

194. Vanilla Sauce

1-1/4 cup milk
1/2 vanilla bean
1 tbsp. raw sugar
1/2 tsp. cornstarch
1 egg
8 tbsp. cream (opt.)

Prepare like Vanilla Cream in recipe No. 184. Beat cream stiffly and fold in.

195. Almond Milk Sauce

1-3/4 cups milk
2 oz. shelled, ground almonds
1-1/2 oz. cane or raw sugar
1 tbsp. cornstarch
2 tbsp. water

Bring milk to a boil and add almonds and sugar. Blend cornstarch and water and stir into the boiling milk. Mix this sauce well.

196. Rose Hip Sauce

2-1/2 oz. rose hip puree or concentrate
4/5 cup water or grape juice
2-1/2 oz. cane sugar
A few drops lemon juice (opt.)

Make rose hip puree by boiling about 1 oz. dried hips in 3-1/2–4 oz. water, and forcing through a sieve. Bring puree, juice, and sugar to a boil. Add lemon juice just before serving.

197. Semolina Mold

5-1/2 oz. semolina
1-1/2 qt. milk
1 pinch salt
2-3 tbsp. raw sugar

1 lemon peel, grated
1 egg, beaten
1-1/2 oz. shelled, ground almonds
1 oz. raisins

Cook semolina in milk, salt and lemon peel to a porridge. Add sugar last. Blend egg, almonds and raisins with the prepared puree and pour into a ring mold. Let cool, rinse mold with cold watcr, tilt on scrving dish. Pour syrup ovcr it. Serve with raspberry syrup.

198. Lemon Rice Pudding

3-1/2 cups water
Juice of 1 lemon
Diced lemon peel
1 pinch salt
5-1/2 oz. raw sugar or honey
5-1/2 oz. rice
4/5 cup cream

Bring water, juice, peel, salt and honey to a boil. Add rice and cook 30 minutes, let cool, fold in the whipped cream and pour into a pudding mold that has been rinsed with cold water. Chill.

199. Almond Blancmange

1 qt. milk
1 lemon peel, grated
1 cup milk
4 oz. cornstarch
1 pinch salt
1 tbsp. raw sugar
3 oz. shelled, ground almonds
2 eggs

Bring milk and lemon peel to a boil. Blend cornstarch with milk and salt, add, and cook 5 min. Take off the flame. Beat sugar, almonds and eggs and add to the milk, stirring rapidly all the while. Pour into a rinsed pudding mold. Chill. Serve with raspberry syrup.

200. Red Grits

3 cups currant, raspberry, or strawberry juice
1 cup red grape juice
2-1/2 oz. semolina
1 tbsp. cornstarch

Bring berry and grape juice to a boil. Make a paste of semolina and cornstarch. Stir into the hot juices and cook 10 minutes. Pour into a cold-rinsed ring mold and chill. Serve with Vanilla Sauce, recipe No. 205.

201. Cottage Cheese Pudding

1-1/2 oz. butter
4 tbsp. flour
1-1/3 cup hot milk
18 oz. cottage cheese
2 eggs
2-1/2 oz. cane or raw sugar
1-1/2 oz. raisins
Grated lemon peel
4 tbsp. cream

Sauté flour in butter. Add milk and boil a few minutes. Mix remaining ingredients with the thickened milk, pour into a pudding mold and bake 30-40 minutes at 350 degrees.

202. Oat Biscuits

7 oz. rolled oats
4 oz. butter
1 egg
9 oz. cane sugar
Vanilla sugar
4 oz. flour
1 egg yolk

Brown oats lightly in butter. Beat egg and sugar until frothy, add to flour and work into a soft dough together with the oats. Roll out the dough to about 1/8 in. thick, cut out biscuits, brush with egg yolk, and bake in an oven at 350 degrees until golden.

203. Swabian Biscuits

5-1/2 oz. butter
9 oz. raw sugar
4 oz. toasted, finely ground hazelnuts
2-1/2 cups whole wheat flour
1-2 eggs
Juice and peel of one lemon
1 pinch cinnamon
1 pinch salt
1 egg yolk

Beat butter and sugar until frothy. Work remaining ingredients into a soft dough and allow to stand 1 hour in a cool place. Roll out dough to about 1/8 in. thick, carve out shapes at will, brush with egg yolk, and bake at 350 degrees.

VII.
Menu Suggestions

These menus are arranged according to various consistencies (see "Diets," page 33).

Juice Form (Diet II)

For special adaptations, see Diet II A, B, C, pages 34-37.

Bed-Juice Day or a Fruit Juice Fast Day

Strict Form: 21 oz. juice

8 a.m.: 7 oz. fresh unsweetened fruit juice—grapefruit, orange, tangerine, berry, peach, melon, etc.; possibly substitute 1/3 cereal puree for the juice

12:30 p.m.: 7 oz. fruit juice (as above) or 7 oz. vegetable juice, fresh, with a few drops of lemon juice—carrots, tomatoes, spinach, beets, mixed or plain

6 p.m.: 7 oz. fruit juice as at 8 a.m.

Prerequisites: Strict bed rest, weight and urine checks in 24 hours. Fast only for 1-3 days, unless under a doctor's supervision.

If there is strong thirst or the amount of urine is insufficient [less than 800 cc. (24 oz.) in 24 hours], 1-3 cups (5-1/2 oz. per cup) rose hip or other tea can be added.

Mild Form: 28 oz. juice

8 a.m.:	7 oz. fruit juice
12 p.m.:	7 oz. mixed or plain vegetable juice
4 p.m.:	7 oz. fruit juice (different juice than at 8 a.m.)
8 p.m.:	5½–7 oz. carrot or tomato juice

Prerequisites: Duration and application as in the Strict Diet.

Full Juice Day

Breakfast: 7 oz. fruit juice (If physician prescribes, add cereal puree or cream, or agar-agar.)
5½ oz. almond or soybean milk, or yogurt
Possibly 1 cup rose hip tea with honey

Lunch: 7 oz. fruit juice
5½ oz. almond or sesame milk, or yogurt
5½ oz. different kinds of plain vegetable juice or mixed from 2-3 kinds

Dinner: 7 oz. fruit juice
5½ oz. almond milk or yogurt

If a completely fat-free diet is necessary, buttermilk, skimmed yogurt, or whey can be substituted for the milk.

Pureed Form (Diet III)

Raw Food Day, pureed

Breakfast: 7 oz. muesli blended, or strained through a sieve
5½ oz. fruit juice
5½ oz. almond milk
1 cup tea

Lunch: 7 oz. fruit juice
5½ oz. almond milk
Mixed raw vegetables—tomatoes, Boston lettuce, carrots

Dinner: Like breakfast

Raw Food Day with Addition, pureed

Breakfast and Dinner: See pureed Raw Food Day

Lunch: 5½ oz. fruit juice
5½ oz. almond milk
5½ oz. vegetable juice or mixed raw vegetables—tomatoes, Boston lettuce, celery root
7 oz. vegetable bouillon
Mashed potatoes

Transitional Diet, pureed

Breakfast: 9 oz. blended muesli
5½ oz. fruit juice
1 cup herb tea or milk or yogurt
1 piece crisp bread or whole wheat zwieback

Lunch: 5½ oz. fruit juice
5½ oz. mixed raw vegetables
Cooked Dishes: green rye soup, strained
chopped Romaine lettuce
mashed potatoes

Dinner: 9 oz. muesli, blended
Cooked dishes: grain soup
Herb tea

Transition Diet (Diet IV)

Raw Food Day, refined

Breakfast: Muesli, possibly strained
5½ oz. almond milk or grated almonds or pine kernels
5½ oz. fruit juice, possibly rose hip tea

Lunch: 5½ oz. fruit juice or finely crushed fruit (berries, peaches, bananas, etc.)
Raw Vegetables: finely grated carrots, chopped zucchini, chopped Boston lettuce
Almond milk or pine kernels

Dinner: Same as breakfast

Raw Food Day with Addition, refined

Breakfast and Dinner: See Raw Food Day, refined
Possibly add 1 piece of crisp bread

Lunch: 5½ oz. fruit juice or finely crushed fruit
Raw Vegetables: finely grated white radish
Cooked Dishes: finely chopped spinach and tomatoes
7 oz. vegetable bouillon
bouillon potatoes

Transitional Diet, refined

Breakfast: 9 oz. muesli

Dinner: 5½ oz. fruit juice
1 cup herb tea or milk or yogurt
1 piece crisp bread with butter

Lunch: 5½ oz. fruit juice or finely crushed fruit
Raw Vegetables: finely grated salsify, finely chopped endive, finely chopped tomatoes
Cooked Dishes: strained potato soup
finely chopped fennel
risotto

Different Types of Maintenance Diet (Diet V)

Fruit Fast

A Fruit Fast can replace a bed-juice-only day, if, instead of a strictly protective fiber-free diet, a change in metabolism and stimulation with cellulose is desired. Since a Fruit Fast gives a stronger sense of satisfaction, such a diet is possible without complete rest and can be carried out longer. However, the effect of the juice fast is more intense.

A Fruit Fast is advisable in the case of intestinal sluggishness (apple, banana, or blueberry day) and constipation in the lower abdomen. It can be taken for 1-5 days, longer, if prescribed by a physician. Also good as a reducing diet.

Daily Menu: 7-9 oz. washed, fresh, completely ripe, and unsweetened fruit, twice daily.

Special Fruit Days:

Apple day: 1 large apple, finely grated, 5-6 times daily, for acute gastroenteritis with diarrhea.

Strawberry day: 7-9 oz. very ripe, unsweetened strawberries, 3-4 times daily.

Blueberry day: 7-9 oz. blueberries, 3 times daily. Slightly constipating, disinfecting.

Blackberry day: 7-9-11 oz. blackberries, 3 times daily. Especially rich in natural sugar and vitamin C, easily digestible and nourishing.

Currant day: 7-9 oz. currants, 3/4 red and yellow, 1/3 black currants, 3 times daily. Rich in vitamin C. Especially refreshing and thirst-quenching for liver patients.

Persimmon day: 2 small or 1 large persimmon, 4 times daily. Rich in vitamins C and B, very nourishing.

Grape day: (A well-known cure): 27-35 oz. grapes, divided

into 4-5 servings a day. Wash well, and disinfect from remains of sprays. Eat fruit whole. Low in vitamins, but especially nourishing because of the high amount of fruit sugar which is easily absorbed. Protects the liver. Seeds stimulate the intestine. Duration 1-2 weeks; can be carried out for up to 6 weeks, if prescribed by a doctor.

Fig day: 7 oz. fresh figs, 3 times daily. Stimulates intestines, nourishing. 1 day at most.

Raw Food Day, normal

Breakfast: Muesli
Fruit (all fruits, except apricots and prunes)
Pine kernels, hazelnuts, almonds

Lunch: Fruit
Raw Vegetables: cauliflower, tomatoes, Romaine lettuce
Pine kernels, hazelnuts, almonds

Dinner: Same as for breakfast

Raw Food Diet with Addition, normal

Breakfast and Dinner: See Raw Food Day, normal
Possibly add 1 slice crispbread

Lunch: Fruit
Raw Vegetables: Chinese cabbage, beets
Almonds, hazelnuts
Cooked Dishes: zucchini,
7 oz. vegetable bouillon, baked potatoes

Transitional Diet, normal

Breakfast: 9 oz. muesli
Dinner: Fruit
1 cup herb tea or milk or yogurt
1 slice whole grain bread with health food store vegetable fat or butter

Lunch: Fruit
Raw Vegetables: cress, cucumbers, carrots
Cooked Dishes: vegetable bouillon,
rice pudding with tomatoes

Menu for 1 Week of a Maintenance Diet

1st day
Breakfast: 9 oz. muesli
1-2 slices whole-grain bread
About ½ oz. butter
Possibly honey or cottage cheese
Fruit
Herb tea

Lunch: Fruit
Raw Vegetables: celery root, dandelion, Boston lettuce
Cooked Dishes: beets, potatoes with cottage cheese, pear compote

Dinner: Yogurt with fruit salad or muesli
Sandwiches
or brown rice and Boston lettuce
or groat porridge with cream

Breakfast and dinner of the following days are the same as on the first day.

2nd day
Lunch: Fruit
Raw Vegetables: salsify, endive
Cooked Dishes: cream of rice soup
tomato halves with scrambled egg
millotto

3rd day
Lunch: Fruit
Raw Vegetables: beets, white cabbage, Boston lettuce
Cooked Dishes: artichokes with butter sauce
Swiss chard with tomatoes
mashed potatoes, II

4th day
Lunch: Fruit
Raw Vegetables: cauliflower, tomatoes, Boston lettuce
Cooked Dishes: carrots
spinach, mini gnocchi
Strawberries in lemon juice

5th day
Lunch: Fruit
Raw Vegetables: white radish, spinach, Boston lettuce
Cooked Dishes: tomato soup
Chinese peas
cream potatoes

6th day
Lunch: Fruit
Raw Vegetables: fennel, carrots, Boston lettuce
Cooked Dishes: Romaine lettuce
rice Creole
junket with raspberries

7th day
Lunch: Fruit
Raw Vegetables: kohlrabi, tomatoes, Boston lettuce
Cooked Dishes: zucchini, polenta, apple cream

VIII. Summary of Foods for Various Digestive Ailments

1. Soothing Disinfectants for Gastroenteritis (see page 19 and Diet II A, page 34)

Whole-grain puree, plain or mixed with fresh juices, agar-agar, barley, brown rice. Kaolin (used internally) between meals mixed with water or a soothing herb tea. Potato juice, raw cabbage juice, and certified milk in swallows. Absolutely fresh cream, skimmed, salt-free cheese. Whey cheese, fresh (not sour) buttermilk, whey, junket, camomile tea.

2. Stimulants for Appetite and Gastric Juices (see page 24 and Diet II C, page 37)

Yeast products, vegetable seasoning, sea salt instead of table salt, and soybean seasoning. Vegetable bouillon (vegetable bouillon cubes), cottage cheese and mild cheeses with herbs. Herbs: marjoram, tarragon, dill, anise. Bitter vegetables: escarole, chicory. Raw vegetable juices seasoned with herbs. If juices cannot be extracted at home, natural pure vegetable juices are available in bottles. Whole-grain sourdough breads, cereal grains and flakes, nuts, raisins, berries, citrus fruits, sour apples, bitter tea, centaury tea.

3. Stimulants for the Intestine when Constipated (see page 43)

Whole-grain dishes from cracked grains (groats), sprouted grains, whole-grain bread. Cereal purees with a slightly laxative effect, such as linseed, ground or whole (cooked to puree with water), fresh fruit, fresh vegetables (green), dried fruit (especially figs, prunes, pears), rhubarb, yogurt, sour milk, whey, sauerkraut or sauerkraut water, sourdough breads.

4. Congestive Effect for Diarrhea
(see Diet II C)

Apples, bananas, blueberry juice, kaolin, carob meal, rice puree, rice flour, rice grains, blackberry leaf tea.

5. For Preventing Flatulence
(see page 29)

Kaolin. Yogurt, buttermilk, whey, anti-flatulent tea (fennel, caraway seed, anise). Linseed puree. Avoid cooked cabbage (use raw or as juice instead), sweets, and sweet milk.

6. Restorative and Convalescent Diet

Minerals, enzymes, vitamins: sea salt, whole grain, all fresh vegetables (whole or in juice form) and fruit, sea buckthorn, wild herb extracts (stinging nettle, watercress, birch, etc.), sprouted grains.

High-quality sugar and starches: Whole-grain flour, flakes, groats, bread, wheat germ or sprouted wheat, whole-grain rusks, pumpernickel, crispbread, sourdough bread, honey, fruit concentrate, natural, unfiltered fruit juices, grape juice, possibly grape sugar, raw sugar, all sweet types of fruit, carrots, beets.

High-quality fat: Cold-pressed sunflower seed, linseed, poppy seed, and wheat germ oils, grade A and uncolored. Fresh butter and cream, vegetable fats as sandwich spread. Pine kernels, almonds, Brazil nuts, and other types of nuts. Sesame seed products.

High-quality protein: (lactovegetal): soybean products (sandwich spread, flour, flakes), almond and hazelnut products (puree, milk, sandwich spreads), sesame seed products. Sour milk, buttermilk, yogurt. Whey. Junket, skim milk, certified milk, cottage cheese with herbs, salt, or honey. Cream cheese. Salt-free cheese. Whey cheese. Raw, fresh egg beaten with fruit juice or in soup. (For diet tables, see page 34).

Diets for Gastrointestinal Patients

I. Fast (page 34)

27-35 oz. herb tea (5-6 glasses, 5-1/2 oz. each). Types of tea: camomile—linden flowers—peppermint—rose hip—blueberry leaf—blackberry leaf—strawberry leaf—linseed—wormwood—Mixed herb teas: anti-flatulent tea, bitter tea. (For use and preparation of different teas, see recipes, pages 46-47).

Tea Fast includes bedrest with uniform warmth, until acute symptoms disappear. Duration according to doctor's prescription.

II. Juice Diet (pp. 48-49)

Fruit

All fresh fruit juices, plain or mixed with cream or 1/3 cereal puree, or with almond milk, crushed apple or banana, or agar-agar jelly.

Vegetables

Raw: All types of juices, mixed with cream or 1/3 puree, or plain, from a juice press or centrifuge. Cooked: homemade ("natural") vegetable bouillon.

Sugars

Honey dissolved in tea and juices, dissolved fruit sugar, dissolved fruit concentrate.

Starches (grain, potatoes)

Cereal purees: linseed, barley, oats, rice, wheat*: 1/3 mixed with juices or plain.

*Patients with Herter's disease should not use grain containing gluten (wheat, rye, barley, oats).

Fats

Cold-pressed vegetable oils (linseed, sunflower seed, olive oils). Use fresh cream moderately.

Protein

Vegetable: almond, soybean, sesame seed milk, raw vegetable juices. Animal: milk, yogurt, kefir, buttermilk, whey, beaten egg yolk (occasionally).

Beverages

Fresh fruit and vegetable juices, natural vegetable bouillon. All types of milk: almond, soybean, sesame seed milk. Herb teas: (See recipes) depending on individual need. Diluted fruit concentrate, non-carbonated mineral water.

Seasonings

Sea salt in vegetable bouillon and purees.

III. Pureed Diet (pp. 38-39)

Fruit

II, III + grapes (wash well), regular and blended Bircher muesli. II + all fruit, mixed in blender, according to individual need, carefully selected, high-quality, organically grown ripe fruit (avoid pesticides). Cooked: strained compote, slightly sweetened.

Vegetables

II + Raw: pureed, blended. Cooked: all types, strained. No cabbages in the beginning, but later, if allowed.

Sugars

As in II. (Mixed in fruit puree and meusli.)

Starches (grain, potatoes)

Whole-grain flakes in muesli or milk. Grain soups. Porridge of coarsely ground whole grain. Crispbread D, well chewed. Mashed or whole potatoes.

Fats

Like II + butter, nutbutter, oleomargarine, use moderately.

Protein

II + vegetable: hazelnut and almond puree, sesame seed, soybean in dessert cream, sandwich spread, flakes, milk. Animal: cottage cheese, whey, milkshakes, junket.

Beverages

Like II.

Seasonings

Like II. Possibly mild herbs.

IV. Transition Diet (Convalescence) (pp. 41-42)

Fruit

II, III + grapes (wash well), regular Bircher muesli or with yogurt or cream.

Vegetables

II, III + Raw: minced, with oil, lemon, cream, herbs. Cooked: all kinds, steamed. Selection depends on digestibility.

Sugars

Like II + raw sugar.

Starches (grain, potatoes)

Crispbreads H and D, pumpernickel, whole-grain breads,

wheat germ, sprouted grains, rice, corn, millet. Porridge of coarsely ground or cracked grains.* All potato dishes.

Fats

Like II + III.

Protein

II, III + all types of milk (vegetable and animal), whole grains,* rarely egg dishes, very mild cheeses.

Beverages

Like II + organic apple juice, pasteurized grape juice, frozen juices (do not drink ice cold, drink slowly).

Seasonings

Like II + fresh kitchen herbs, rosemary, thyme, dill, lovage, marjoram, tarragon, lemon balm, vegetable and yeast extracts.

V. Maintenance Diet For Preventing Illness (pp. 43-44)

Fruit

I, II, III + Raw: all ripe fresh fruit, well chewed. Cooked: compote as an exception.

Vegetables

II, III, IV + Raw and Cooked: all vegetables, well chewed. Organically grown if possible, well cleaned; save cooking water; do not reheat. Use fresh butter or oil for steaming or serving.

Sugars

Like IV. White sugar as an exception only. Avoid chocolate and candy completely.

*See footnote, page 134.

Starches

Whole-grain breads, groat porridge, sprouted wheat, all grain dishes, whole-grain flours, whole-grain noodles, etc.*

Fats

Like II + III + occasional servings of fried or baked foods, heated fats. No hard fats.

Protein

Like IV + cottage cheese-fruit cream desserts, different types of mild cheeses, herbed cottage cheese, eggs (two per week). Meat: up to two times weekly, if desired.

Beverages

Like II-IV. No alcohol, coffee, or black tea.

Seasonings

Like IV, to taste. Also some nutmeg, paprika.

Special Effects of Certain Foods

Stimulate Gastric Juices and Appetite

Fruit

Citrus fruit, ripe, grapes (not too sweet), all berries, melons, sweet ripe peaches, plums, cherries.

Vegetables

All raw vegetables, chewed well, particularly raw and cooked spinach, cress, and sauerkraut.

Sugars

Honey and fruit concentrate.

*See footnote, page 134.

Starches (grain, potatoes)

Sprouted grains, whole grains, groats, grits, whole-grain breads (sour dough). Baked and boiled potatoes.

Fats

Small amount of cold-pressed vegetable oils.

Protein

Yogurt, kefir, buttermilk, fruit milk (blended cold), sour milk, herb cheese and cottage cheese, caraway seed cheese, etc.

Beverages

Bitter tea, peppermint tea, centaury tea, rose hip tea, vegetable bouillon, fresh juices, apple juice and pasteurized grape juice, yogurt, buttermilk, juniper berry juice (by spoonfuls, pasteurized).

Seasonings

Only in diets III-V. Sea salt, vegetable and yeast extracts, a little paprika, nutmeg, fresh or dried kitchen herbs: rosemary, dill, tarragon, marjoram, thyme, mint balm, lovage.

Calming Gastric Juices

Fruit

Apples, bananas, juices plus 1/3 puree or jelly, sweet, mild grape juice.

Vegetables

Raw juices + 1 tbsp. cream + 1/3 puree + raw potato juice. Especially carrots, beets, and cabbage, blended or as juice.

Sugars

Honey and fruit concentrate.

Starches (grain, potatoes)

Rice, barley, oats puree (strained, salt-free), rolled grain and whole-grain flour (pureed with milk or water); crispbread, mashed potatoes and raw potato juice.

Fats

Small amounts of almond milk, cream and vegetable oil.

Protein

Sweet milk, certified milk, almond milk, junket, cottage cheese, natural mild soft cheeses (Gervais).

Beverages

Camomile, linseed, and linden flower teas, sweet milk, fresh juices diluted with noncarbonated mineral water.

Seasonings

Salt-free, natural, without seasonings.

Intestinally Stimulating (Against Constipation)

Fruit

Citrus fruit, berries, grapes, rhubarb, ripe pitted fruit, dried fruit (figs, prunes).

Vegetables

All raw and cooked vegetables, chewed well.

Sugars

Honey and fruit concentrate, date sugar.

Starches (grain, potatoes)

Sprouted whole grain, whole-grain breads, groats, grits, linseed puree. Boiled and baked potatoes.

Fats

Small amount of cold-pressed vegetable oils.

Protein

As under "Stimulates Gastric Juices."

Beverages

Linseed tea, yogurt, fresh juices, mineral water (containing magnesium).

Seasonings

Buckthorn bark, Cascara Sagrada or chittam bark (as seasoning or tea, in small doses), sea salt.

Settles Intestinal Activity (Against Diarrhea and Flatulence)

Fruits

Blueberry compote (fresh and dried blueberries), blueberry juice or tea, strawberries, black currants, grated apples, bananas.

Vegetables

Juice of raw vegetables (no spinach or cabbages), pureed cooked vegetables (without spinach).

Sugars

None.

Starches (grain, potatoes)

As under "Settles Gastric Juices."

Fats

As under "Settles Gastric Juices."

Protein

As under "Settles Gastric Juices."

Beverages

Blackberry leaf tea, dried blueberries (by boiling down), lemon balm tea, camomile tea, orange blossom tea, peppermint tea, anti-flatulence tea (from caraway seed, fennel, anise).

Seasonings

Dried blueberries.